Complete Guide to Landmine Training

David Otey, CSCS
Joe Drake, MS, CSCS

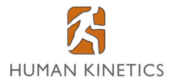

HUMAN KINETICS

Library of Congress Cataloging-in-Publication Data

Names: Otey, David, 1988- author. | Drake, Joe, 1987- author.
Title: Complete guide to landmine training / David Otey, Joe Drake.
Description: Champaign, IL : Human Kinetics, [2026] | Includes
   bibliographical references.
Identifiers: LCCN 2024044028 (print) | LCCN 2024044029 (ebook) | ISBN
   9781718217942 (paperback) | ISBN 9781718217959 (epub) | ISBN
   9781718217966 (pdf)
Subjects: LCSH: Weight training--Equipment and supplies. |
   Exercise--Equipment and supplies. | Isometric exercise.
Classification: LCC GV543 .O84 2026 (print) | LCC GV543 (ebook) | DDC
   613.7/1--dc23/eng/20241212
LC record available at https://lccn.loc.gov/2024044028
LC ebook record available at https://lccn.loc.gov/2024044029

ISBN: 978-1-7182-1794-2 (print)

This publication is written and published to provide accurate and authoritative information relevant to the subject matter presented. It is published and sold with the understanding that the author and publisher are not engaged in rendering legal, medical, or other professional services by reason of their authorship or publication of this work. If medical or other expert assistance is required, the services of a competent professional person should be sought.

The web addresses cited in this text were current as of September 2024, unless otherwise noted.

Senior Acquisitions Editor: Michelle Earle; **Developmental Editor:** Anne Hall; **Managing Editor:** Kevin Matz; **Copyeditor:** Coker Publishing Services; **Proofreader:** Mary Elisabeth Frediani; **Permissions Manager:** Laurel Mitchell; **Graphic Designer:** Dawn Sills; **Cover Designer** Keri Evans; **Cover Design Specialist:** Susan Rothermel Allen; **Photographs (cover and interior):** CDRVisuals/© Human Kinetics unless otherwise noted; **Photo Asset Manager:** Laura Fitch; **Photo Production Specialist:** Amy M. Rose; **Photo Production Manager:** Jason Allen; **Senior Art Manager:** Kelly Hendren; **Printer:** Versa Press

We thank Axios Fitness in Boca Raton, Florida, for assistance in providing the location for the photo shoot for this book.

Human Kinetics books are available at special discounts for bulk purchase. Special editions or book excerpts can also be created to specification. For details, contact the Special Sales Manager at Human Kinetics.

Printed in the United States of America   10   9   8   7   6   5   4   3   2   1

The paper in this book is certified under a sustainable forestry program.

Human Kinetics
1607 N. Market Street
Champaign, IL 61820
USA

United States and International
Website: **US.HumanKinetics.com**
Email: info@hkusa.com
Phone: 1-800-747-4457

Canada
Website: **Canada.HumanKinetics.com**
Email: info@hkcanada.com

E8932

Complete Guide to Landmine Training

Contents

Exercise Finder   vii

Foreword by Bert Sorin from Sorinex   xi

Introduction: Strength for the Masses   xiii

PART I   THE SCIENCE OF LANDMINE TRAINING

1 Foundations of Landmine Training   **3**

2 Setup, Attachments, and Safety   **21**

PART II   LANDMINE EXERCISES

3 Upper Body Exercises   **37**
- Upper Pushing Exercises   38
- Upper Pulling Exercises   64
- Upper Body Accessory Exercises   75

4 Lower Body Exercises   **81**
- Squatting Exercises   82
- Lunge Exercises   98
- Hinge Exercises   122
- Lower Body Accessory Exercises   138

5 Full Body Exercises   **143**

6 Core Exercises   **173**

PART III LANDMINE PROGRAMS

7   Foundations of Program Design   **203**

8   Total Body Conditioning   **211**

9   Advanced Conditioning   **223**

10   Hypertrophy Training   **231**

11   Strength Development   **239**

12   Power Training   **247**

References   253

About the Authors   255

Earn Continuing Education Credits/Units   258

Exercise Finder

Chapter 3: Upper Body Exercises

Upper Pushing Exercises

Half-Kneeling Lateral Press	52
Half-Kneeling Single-Arm Press	50
Kneeling Landmine Press	48
Rollout Push-Up	56
Rotational Single-Arm Press	46
Seated Single-Arm Press	54
Single-Arm Floor Press	60
Single-Arm Press	42
Single-Arm Z-Press	58
Staggered Single-Arm Press	44
Standing Chest Fly	62
Standing Shoulder-to-Shoulder Press	40
Standing Two-Arm Landmine Press	38

Upper Pulling Exercises

Meadows Row	70
Variation: Staggered Meadows Row	72
Single-Leg RDL Row	74
Staggered Single-Arm Row	68
Two-Handed Landmine Row (Prison Row)	64
Variation: T-Bar Row	66

Upper Body Accessory Exercises

Concentration Curl	78
Lateral Raise	77
Mixed-Grip Curl	79
Upright Row	75

Chapter 4: Lower Body Exercises

Squatting Exercises

Hack Squat	88
Kickstand Squat	92
Landmine Goblet Squat	82
Variation: Heels-Elevated Squat	84
Offset Squat	86
Offset Surfer Squat	90
Sissy Squat	94
Squat with Sidestep	96

Lunge Exercises

Angled Landmine Reverse Lunge	112
Bottom-Loaded Reverse Lunge	110
Bulgarian Split Squat	120
Lateral Lunge	100
Rear Foot Elevated (RFE) Split Squat	118
Split Squat	114
Variation: Front Foot Elevated (FFE) Split Squat	116
Static Lateral Lunge	98
Top-Loaded Reverse Lunge	102
Variation: Step-Through Reverse Lunge	104
Variation: Elevated Reverse Lunge	106
Variation: Overhead Reverse Lunge	108

Hinge Exercises

Adductor RDL	126
Forward-Facing RDL	122
Kneeling Hip Extension	134
Landmine Sumo Deadlift	136
Rear-Facing RDL	124
Single-Leg RDL	132
Staggered RDL	128
Stepping RDL	130

Lower Body Accessory Exercises

Staggered Calf Raise	140
Standing Calf Raise	138

Chapter 5: Full Body Exercises

Kneeling Push Press	150
Landmine Hang Clean	152
Landmine Thruster	144
Lateral Snatch	170
Push Press	166
Reverse Lunge Thruster	158
Rotational RDL-to-Press	162
Rotational Squat-to-Press	160
Single-Arm Clean	154
Single-Leg RDL-to-Row	156
Split Jerk	168
Squat Hold Press	148
Squat Jump	146
Step-Through Press	164

Chapter 6: Core Exercises

Bear Position Body Saw	196
Bear Position Ticktock	194
Bent Press	199
Landmine Anchored Deadbug	176
Landmine Anchored Leg Lift	180
Landmine Anchored Reverse Crunch	178
Variation: Landmine Bear Crawl	197
Landmine March	174
Landmine Rollout	192
Landmine Straight-Leg Sit-Up	182
Offset Core Rotations	186
Rainbows	188
Tall Kneeling Offset Rotations	190
Ticktocks	184
Variation: Windmills	198

Foreword

They say necessity is the mother of invention, and the best inventions are generally the simple ones. The landmine is simple: an anchor point, a universal joint, and a coupling sleeve. Just three components. Yet the movements and the results it produces are anything but simple. While my late father, Richard Sorin, and I invented the modern-day landmine, we left plenty of room for exploration in angled barbell training. Innovators like David Otey have dedicated their time and passion to unlocking the full potential of this incredibly effective training tool.

In 2000, as I trained for a hopeful spot on the U.S. Olympic team in the hammer throw, I felt a bit undersized. I felt like I needed an edge. I decided to explore a corner of my training that would integrate barbell movements with the functional capacity to produce force in a new vector. Suddenly, the landmine was born. We named it the *landmine* because my father and I believed it would enhance explosiveness at ground level. The name may have been a bit cheeky, but it stuck. The rotational twist quickly became the foundational movement, but we soon began to explore other possibilities.

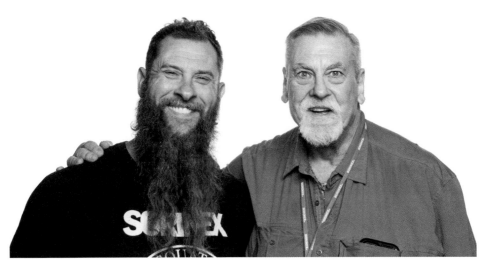

Bert and Richard "Pops" Sorin
Courtesy of SORINEX.

Over the next few years, landmine training evolved throughout the industry, producing both effective techniques and less effective ones. Just because you can, that doesn't mean you should. However, in training, as in life, the best practices eventually rise to the top. After thousands of repetitions and multiple peer reviews, the best practices began to show themselves. The best movements emerged, and they became staples in the modern human performance industry.

As insightful coaches continue to explore landmine training, they refine techniques, positions, load parameters, and movement intensity. Like all exercises, landmine training has its inherent strengths and weaknesses, making it crucial to understand the physiological effects of each application. What began as a tool has spawned new exercises, which led to further discovery, refinement, and eventually the development of effective training programs.

Complete Guide to Landmine Training covers all of this in a way that both beginners and advanced athletes or coaches can understand, tracing the journey from its origin to its most effective applications for goal-driven training. This book distills years of knowledge on landmine training, detailing when to use it (or not) and clarifying each step along the path to success. No rep has been spared.

While I am proud to have played a part in the landmine's origin, nothing makes me happier than witnessing how David and others have expanded its possibilities. I hope you enjoy *Complete Guide to Landmine Training* and feel inspired to embark on your own strength exploration journey. I know I am.

In strength,
Bert Sorin
President and Co-Owner of Sorinex

Introduction

If strength training is touted as the fountain of youth, then barbells are seen as the holy grail. While barbell work is arguably the best-known way to get brutally strong, the rigid approach most people take can leave gaps in their training. Landmine training bridges this gap to create more accessible training options for those looking for alternative ways of intelligently building strength with free weights.

Spawned from the highest levels of performance training, landmine training has given us an entirely new way to look at using barbells. Its unique design and arced bar path make it the ultimate training tool for learning to control and create rotation—a fundamental skill most people never train. Offering joint-friendly range of motion, enhanced core stability, and safer power movements, the landmine is truly one of the most versatile and underutilized tools in the gym.

Until now.

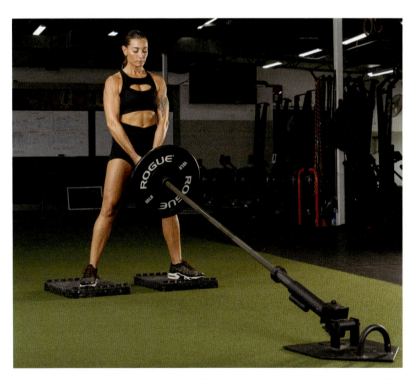

Landmine training provides a different type of stimulus than traditional movements, resulting in a major impact on your body.

The best of the best have been reaping the benefits of landmine training for years, but this book isn't just about training athletes. It's about creating strength for the masses and making barbell training more accessible for all. Whether you're brand new to training or a veteran in the gym, introducing landmine training into your routine will have a major impact on your body and provide a different training stimulus than traditional movements.

What follows is broken down into three sections:

1. **Part I: The Science of Landmine Training.** This section introduces some of the foundational training principles that make landmine training unique. These chapters will level up your understanding of why and how to safely to implement landmine training in your program.

2. **Part II: Landmine Exercises.** This section covers the most effective landmine exercises, divided by region of the body (lower body, upper body, full body, and core). We have categorized the exercises by major movement patterns for flexible programming. Each exercise includes simple step-by-step instructions as well as modifications and coaching tips to make sure you get the most out of every move.

3. **Part III: Landmine Programs.** This section puts it all together by giving you ready-to-use programs to follow. We have provided stand-alone landmine programs for all ability levels and goals. This section also teaches you how to think about landmine programming, giving examples of how to integrate individual exercises into your current training program.

In the pages of this book, you'll find that the landmine not only offers an immense amount of exercise variety but could also be the key to unlocking a new level of strength, performance, and fun in your approach toward training.

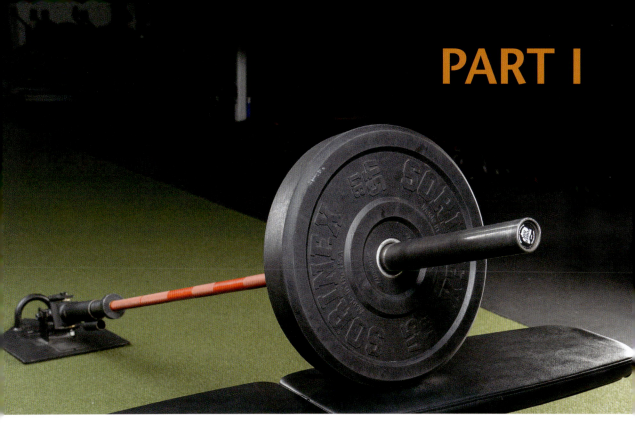

PART I

THE *SCIENCE* OF LANDMINE TRAINING

Currently, the body of research on landmine training is minimal. However, several well-researched scientific training principles support its use as a valid training modality. Part 1 presents some of the science behind landmine training and how you can best use these principles to guide your workouts and maximize results.

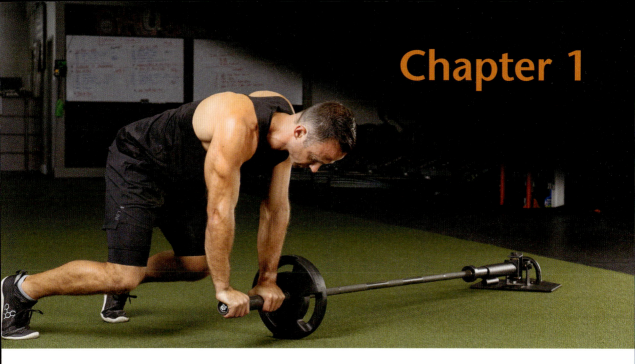

Chapter 1

FOUNDATIONS OF LANDMINE TRAINING

The word is out, and people are catching on—strength training is essential. Research has irrefutably established the benefits of strength training, and interest has been on the rise over the last few decades. It is apparent that most people—if not all—should be lifting. What's often not talked about is what tools might be best for the job. With so many types of equipment available, deciding what to use and how to use it can be a challenging task. This paralysis by analysis means many exercisers never venture outside their comfort zone, and some never get started at all

Many people are looking for ways to continue their pursuit of health and wellness without exacerbating existing injuries. Regardless of whether an exerciser has a long or short training history, they may face physical limitations related to the knees, hips, lower back, and shoulders. These issues may halt training programs that have limited equipment options, but introducing new and versatile alternatives to traditional exercises can provide a new path for people to continue their strength training journey.

Every time you walk into the gym, you have a choice of what equipment to use to best achieve your goals. Although landmine training has been around for a few decades, most gym goers have very little knowledge of the massive training benefits it can offer. This chapter kicks off our journey of changing that for you—arming you with the knowledge and understanding needed to begin using the landmine as an effective training tool.

THE EVOLUTION AND IMPORTANCE OF THE LANDMINE

The need for alternative ways to overload the body in unique positions is at the heart of why the landmine was born. Early uses of the angled barbell setup can be traced back to the golden era of bodybuilding, with athletes like Arnold Schwarzenegger using it for T-bar rows. More recent innovations in landmine training can be traced directly back to Bert Sorin and the legendary company Sorinex. With the help of his father, the late great Richard "Pops" Sorin, Bert invented the landmine joint attachment as a way to better train for the hammer throw as he prepared for the 2000 Olympic Trials. He was looking for a way to bridge the gap between traditional squat and rotary motions that were available with other pieces of equipment to improve explosion from the ground up—hence the "landmine" was born. This type of exploration in the weight room is tied closely to the field of biomechanics, which is the study of human movement and forces. In the weight room, these forces are often the tools and weights we choose to use.

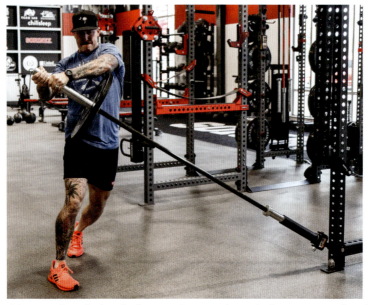

The Sorins' innovations in landmine equipment have led to greater developments in strength training techniques for the whole body.
Courtesy of SORINEX.

EXERCISE MECHANICS AND EQUIPMENT

Leverage and torque are the building blocks of strength training. *Leverage* refers to the mechanical advantage gained by using a lever to apply force. *Torque* can be defined as a rotational force. Our body's muscles and joints use torque to drive movement and are the main things we manipulate in the gym when strength training. You might think you are pulling the dumbbell into your body when performing a dumbbell bent-over row, but the movement is actually a combination of rotational forces (torque) being applied on the shoulder and elbow joints simultaneously to row the dumbbell.

To set the stage for understanding both strength training and the landmine as a tool, it's important to note that there are three types of lever systems (see figure 1.1).

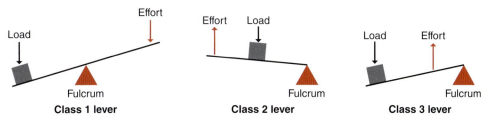

Figure 1.1   Visual examples of first-, second-, and third-class levers.

Although our body uses a few first- and second-class levers to perform certain movements, most of the body's movements are driven by third-class levers (see figure 1.2). Movement with third-class levers is the least efficient of the three types because it requires our muscles to exert greater effort and force. However, it offers some important advantages, such as the potential for larger movements and greater speed of movement.

Understanding a little bit of biomechanics matters because the

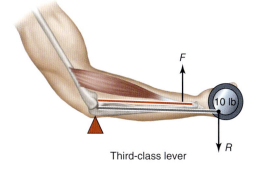

Figure 1.2   The third-class lever system in the elbow, where the forces our muscles exert (F) to overcome the resistance created by the dumbbell (R) are close to the axis of rotation at the joint.

placement of weight in relation to the body can directly affect muscle recruitment and an exercise's impact. The torque level of an exercise can also directly affect how stress is distributed between the soft tissue and joint structures.

With unique pieces of equipment like the landmine, it becomes possible to manipulate training positions and use the concept of torque to our advantage. This means that you can train your body in positions and generate force in certain directions that would not be possible without the landmine. This is the conceptual basis for why landmine training is so prevalent in performance athletics, particularly in activities where the expression of power or rotation is essential. However, the adaptable nature of the landmine is not limited to athletes. It can be a perfect implement for all exercisers, especially those looking to enhance the efficiency of their workouts and to introduce barbell training in a way that may be more accessible for them than traditional barbell lifts.

BENEFITS OF LANDMINE TRAINING

Aside from the physical benefits discussed in this section, the landmine also alleviates the need for large amounts of space and equipment. Because the landmine has a fixed end with a single pivot point, exercisers have 360 degrees of motion and endless opportunities to put torque to use. This means that pushing, pulling, squatting, hinging, lunging, and rotating can all be done in one space with the same piece of equipment. Sometimes called "the corner gym," the landmine offers a variety of training options that require very little equipment to perform and are quick to set up, as you will see in the numerous exercises included in this book. Let's look more closely at the benefits that make this versatile tool a must-have in your strength training arsenal.

Improved Functional Ability

Functional training continues to be one of the most widely debated concepts in the fitness industry—and for good reason. Fitness fads have created confusion around functional training because most fitness enthusiasts assume that a wobble board or unstable surface must be involved for an exercise to be called functional.

The error that most people make is labeling an exercise or method as being *functional* when the term has more to do with the training outcome. In regard to movement, *function* is simply defined as the ability to successfully complete the task at hand. This means that nearly anything can be functional as long as it improves the quality of movement and enhances a desired performance outcome (Siff 2002).

Since the term *function* is specific to the individual and task, perhaps a more useful way of looking at training and how it carries over into life or sport lies in focusing on *functional ability*. This means not just being able to complete a task, but also executing it well and having those skills carry over into other tasks and physical challenges. Ultimately, for most people training is about having physical freedom.

Fitness industry writer and angled barbell pioneer Nick Tumminello (2019) said it best: "Freedom is the absence of constraint. So, having a functional body is about having more physical freedom. This means building an all-around stronger, more adaptable body that's capable of performing at a higher level in any environment—not just inside the gym."

If the goal is physical freedom, then the best place to start is with strength. Building general strength when it comes to squatting, lunging, pushing, pulling, etc. can be done with many types of equipment (e.g., machines, free weights, cables), but not all tools are created equal. Successful performance of activities in the real world requires us to not only generate and absorb forces but also to control (or stabilize) them. The stabilization component of this performance paradigm is what sets the landmine apart as a special tool.

The level of stability required for any exercise can be thought of as existing on a continuum (see figure 1.3). On one end of the continuum are machines that provide maximum external support to the body, like a leg press. The exercises supported by these machines are not just for beginners; they are a great option for anyone who wants to build muscle or strength without being limited by their skill level or ability to maintain stability. However, these types of exercise are often not seen as functional.

On the opposite end are less stable exercises like step-ups, sprinting, and plyometric exercises that demand a high amount of internally generated stability to execute without compromising form or losses in performance. In between are hundreds of exercise variations that feature a mixture of both along the spectrum. Neither end of the spectrum is bad or good; they just result in different outcomes.

Depending on your goals and phase of training, utilizing exercises along the entire continuum can be valuable. However, working in the middle and toward the internal stability end of the continuum can help you learn to better

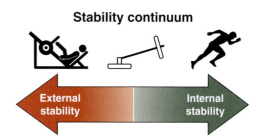

Figure 1.3   All exercises can be placed somewhere on the stability continuum based upon the level of external stability provided by the equipment or position in relation to the internal stability required to successfully complete the movement.

stabilize within your own body. This may be the key to unlocking greater athleticism and transferable strength for many exercisers.

Thankfully, you don't have to (nor should you) choose to live at one end of the spectrum or the other. The landmine is a potential tool for getting the best of both worlds as it offers an opportunity to easily work along the continuum. You can quickly increase or decrease the stability of an exercise based on the movement chosen and the position it's performed in without changing equipment. For example, with the single-leg Romanian deadlift (RDL), the landmine increases external stability (over the pure single-leg alternative) because it acts as an additional point of contact with the ground. This makes it easier to balance and allows you to overload the movement more than you would be able to otherwise to build muscle and strength.

In contrast, the staggered single-arm landmine press requires a much greater level of internal stability throughout the hips, core, and shoulder complex compared to a similar overhead dumbbell press. The long lever of the landmine overhead press creates an immense amount of lateral instability and forces the involvement of many muscle groups to prevent the landmine from shifting side to side (see figure 1.4).

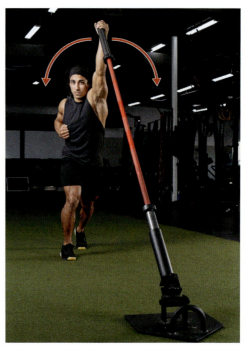

Figure 1.4 In the staggered single-arm landmine press, the entire body must work hard to control the lateral movement and rotation—requiring more internal stability.

It almost always pays to be strong, but once you've achieved a certain level of strength, more doesn't always mean better (depending on your goal or sport). Whether you're a pro athlete seeking to improve performance on the field, just trying to improve your physique, or enhancing your pickleball game, only chasing strength on the stable end of the continuum can get you into trouble over time. Lifting heavy isn't inherently dangerous, but it does require higher levels of skill and technique in training under heavier loads or to failure. It's a skill that takes patience and time, and oftentimes it's a skill that exercisers might not prioritize enough in the pursuit of getting strong. Unless your goals demand absolute maximum strength (most don't), then continuing to train that way may present training risks that outweigh the benefits. Once an exerciser has achieved a certain level of strength on the stable end of the continuum, they might also benefit from working to improve and challenge their strength further down the continuum as well.

From the exercises and workouts in this book, you will see that the landmine can be a great tool for building strength in the gym, adding just the right amount of instability and variation to build a body that's better prepared to tackle life outside the weight room.

Improved Mechanics

Most movement patterns are done through the semicircular motion of third-class levers. The hips and shoulders are ball-and-socket joints that serve as the body's primary movement junctions. To put it simply, they are heavily responsible for generating or controlling almost every movement we do.

Whether you're running, squatting, pushing, pulling, or throwing, the hips and shoulders are the major players, often involving the semicircular motion of the joints (see figure 1.5).

While the hinging motion of the major ball-and-socket joints plays a role in exercises done with traditional free weights, landmine alternatives may allow for a more natural and accessible bar path for common exercises such as the overhead press and squat (see figure 1.6). As the arm or leg moves along the fixed axis of the joint, the end of the joint (distal portion) creates a semicircle. This is the hallmark feature of the landmine—a fixed pivot point with the long lever pivoting around—sort of like your hips and shoulders and their ball-and-socket joints.

With the shoulders and hips being the major drivers of movement, they also tend to be the biggest sources of issues or limitations for many exercisers. The ball-and-socket design provides the potential for a variety of movement in all directions, but when it comes to the human body, nothing works in isolation. Most major movements—pushing, pulling, squat-

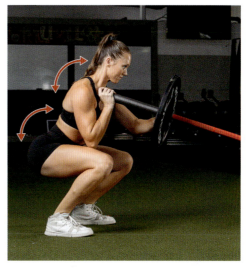

Figure 1.5   A semicircular motion is involved in nearly every movement and exercise that occurs at both the hips and shoulders.

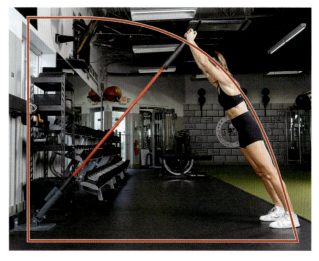

Figure 1.6   The semicircular bar path closely mimics that of our major joints.

ting, etc.—also require various levels of stability (control) and mobility (ability to move) throughout the rest of the body, and this is where the landmine can help.

As you will see described in some of the solutions that follow, the landmine setup can make certain movements more accessible for those who lack the mobility to perform their more traditional exercise counterparts.

More Accessible Overhead Press

Vertical pressing should have a place in most training programs, but direct overhead pressing isn't for everyone. A majority of gym goers lack the thoracic spine mobility, shoulder mobility, and core stability required to effectively press weights directly overhead. Yet nearly everyone still does exercises like the dumbbell press and barbell military press.

Although pressing directly overhead is great, several alternatives offer many of the same benefits. Unfortunately, many gym goers don't know what those alternatives are. The Overhead Clearing Test is a quick screening test that can offer guidance on whether you should press overhead or seek an alternative. Perform the simple overhead clearing test shown in figure 1.7.

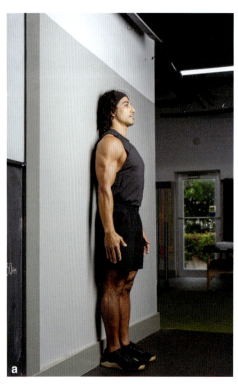 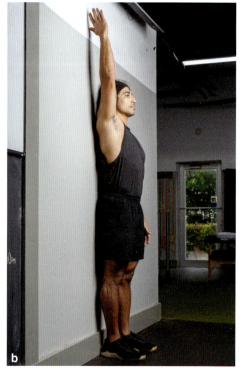

Figure 1.7   The overhead clearing test. *(a)* Stand with your heels, butt, shoulders, and head against the wall. *(b)* Keep your arms straight and slowly raise them up overhead to contact the wall.

If you couldn't bring either arm in contact with the wall without arching your low back, or if you felt a strong pinching sensation in the neck and shoulders, then vertical overhead work might not be your best option right now. The reasons as to why your overhead mobility is restricted are beyond the scope of this book.

Your goal is to find movements and tools that allow you to train safely with the most appropriate movement pattern and intensity, and this is where the landmine shines because of its ability to play between the vertical and horizontal directions. The single-arm landmine press is probably one of the most effective overhead pressing alternatives that you can introduce to continue building overhead position strength. The bar position allows for a more natural motion of the shoulder blade around the rib cage as you press overhead, and because of the slight forward motion of the bar, you aren't limited by mobility and stability issues (see figure 1.8).

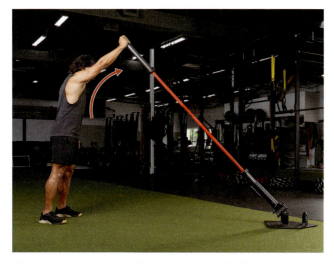

Figure 1.8   The landmine press still offers vertical pressing but without having to go directly overhead and compromise position for those who may have limitations.

The single-arm landmine press also adds the bonus element of core and shoulder stability as the body has to learn to control the long lever of the landmine. The result is the ability to train with intensity overhead but without the unnecessary stress that true vertical pressing, such as with a barbell military press, could cause.

Hinge-Friendly

Hinging refers to hamstring- and glute-focused exercises such as the RDL. The hip hinge is one of the toughest movement patterns to master, but when it comes to creating pain-free movement and physical freedom, it is also one of the most important. Low back and hip pain can create fear of loading the hinge and training it with intensity, but building strength in the hamstrings and glutes can be essential in preventing it. Hinging at the hips is a natural human motion and one of the ways we categorize programming in this book. The key to exercises that focus on hinging is choosing the right exercises, tools, and positions. The landmine can offer some smart alternatives to your hip-dominant training (see figure 1.9).

Based on your setup, you can take advantage of the arc path of the bar to not only alter the range of motion but also to change the direction in which forces are acting on your body and where you place your center of mass. This may allow for some who struggle with traditional RDLs and deadlifting from the ground to effectively train the hinge with intensity and target the muscles involved while minimizing low back strain.

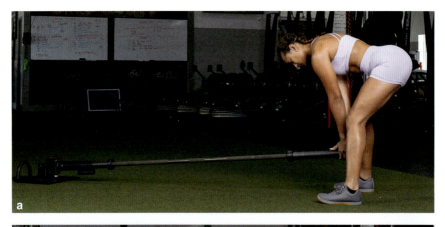

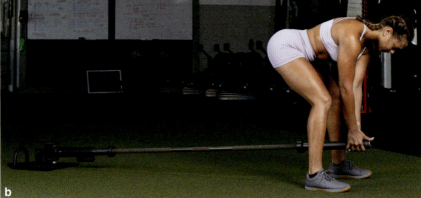

Figure 1.9   For those struggling with hinging, the (*a*) forward-facing landmine RDL and (*b*) rear-facing landmine RDL offer a great alternative by guiding a fixed bar path and aiding in stability of the low back.

The third point of contact that the landmine offers also makes it a superior tool for introducing staggered-stance and hybrid single-leg hinging variations as you look to progress the stability challenge with the hinge without jumping headfirst into pure single-leg stances (see figure 1.10).

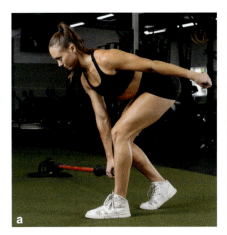 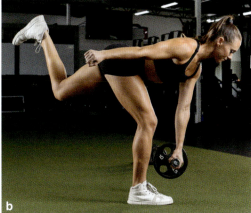

Figure 1.10   Comparison of the *(a)* staggered and *(b)* pure single-leg positions.

The landmine can also be a great tool for learning and executing proper squat technique. The landmine goblet squat gives you no option but to initiate the squat with your hips (i.e., a hinge) because the bar path has both vertical and horizontal components—in other words, it pushes you back and down into position (see figure 1.11). This can be great for anyone looking to build strength in the entire posterior chain (including the mid-back) as well as for those who struggle to "sit back" or who lack the ankle mobility necessary for traditional squatting.

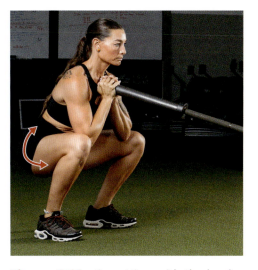

Figure 1.11   Squatting with the landmine can help to put people in better positions because of circular bar path that forces a back and down movement.

Ability to Manipulate Position

The fixed pivot point of the barbell is unique to landmine training and provides the opportunity to place your body in positions and generate forces in directions that would otherwise not be possible with traditional free weights.

For example, with overhead pressing, as discussed earlier, the landmine allows for the creation of a horizontal component to the force generated. This means you not only push it up, but also slightly forward. The landmine also gives us the ability to create a lot of small tweaks in position and body angle with an exercise like the landmine press to make it more or less vertical. The ability to make these small adjustments in leverage and position can be the difference between a pain-free and a painful exercise position.

From an athletic performance standpoint, the landmine is helpful in creating strength that will transfer to the field of play. Very few movements happen in the real world or performance arena without some sort of forward projection of force. Running and walking are both simple but great examples. If you weren't pushing back at an angle (vertically and horizontally) with your feet, then you wouldn't travel forward. This is likely why the landmine became an intuitive training tool for those like Bert Sorin and other athletes looking for greater carryover to the types of forces they needed to generate in competition.

Not every exercise in the gym needs to mimic your sport or desired outcome, but the principle of mechanical specificity states that the more closely it mimics the same movement patterns and direction of forces, then the greater transfer it may have. Better put, being able to manipulate position opens up more possibilities for targeting specific abilities like the forward or even lateral projection of forces that may be hard to replicate with other training tools.

Enhanced Core Training

While core training plays an important role in aesthetics, strength, and performance, it's also one of the most misunderstood areas in fitness. The most common approach for training the core relies on the use of isolated floor exercises like V-ups and bicycle crunches. Isolation training for the core absolutely has value, but most exercises only target a few muscles (e.g., rectus abdominis and external obliques) among the dozens that make up the core.

For the sake of how we present core training throughout the remainder of this book, you can consider nearly every muscle from the knees to the shoulders to be considered part of the core. This view is much broader and includes muscles like the glutes and lats because of the role they play in the two primary functions of this region of the body: the generation and transfer of forces between the hips and shoulders.

Force Transfer

The ability to keep our torso somewhat rigid and appropriately transfer forces between the upper and lower body plays an essential role in nearly all compound lifts and athletic movements. This doesn't mean the torso is *only* meant to remain stiff and resist movement, but it's important that we train it to be the connection point between the upper and lower extremities through integrated core and full body movements—moves that force the lower and upper body to work together.

Research also supports this approach as a more effective method of increasing core activation. A 2013 study published in the *Journal of Strength & Conditioning Research* indicated that activation of the abdominal and lumbar muscles was greatest during exercises that required deltoid and gluteal recruitment (Gottschall et al. 2013). This tends to be greatest when training in positions that require the feet or hands (or both) to be in contact with a fixed surface like the ground. This can be simplified by looking at the difference between a standing cable chop and something like Russian twists. Both are rotational core movements, but the cable chop requires significantly more engagement from the hips and shoulders, which is likely to result in greater core activation.

This describes the majority of exercises you'll find inside this book. The shoulders are engaged in holding the landmine while the hips are engaged in a kneeling or standing position. Many of the movements you will see can initially be taught with core stiffness to emphasize building stability through the core. This is the best place for most people to start when it comes to integrated core training with the landmine, but most moves can also quickly progress to train the core as a force generator as well. Regardless of whether you are looking at the upper body, lower body, or core training exercises in this book, this concept makes the landmine an intuitive tool for training force transfer and integration of the core.

Improved Lateral Stability

Although you get some of the integrated core training benefits mentioned above with traditional strength movements like barbell squats and deadlifts, they often fail to address what's known as the frontal plane (i.e., side-to-side movements). Training the lateral core musculature is an important aspect of improving the performance of activities such as walking, lunging, running, and changing direction. This is because of the demands these activities place on muscles that connect to the hips and help control side-to-side motion. Muscles like the adductors, abductors, obliques, and quadratus lumborum play an increased role in maintaining stability while we are moving. They are still active with traditional lifts, but they are not challenged to control side-to-side forces in the same ways that they may be with tools like the landmine.

Although we can train frontal plane stability through isometric moves like side planks and offset loads, the landmine offers a unique challenge to lateral stability due to its design.

Since the landmine involves a rotating fixed pivot point, as we lift it off the floor into shoulder-racked or overhead positions, the bar can only move side to side. This side-to-side instability is amplified in comparison to other tools because the long lever design means our entire body from the ground up has to work overtime to control the potential torque on the bar.

Rotational Core Training

Just as most training programs lack significant frontal plane core work, the transverse plane (rotational movement) is often neglected yet essential for optimizing performance. Just look at an image of muscular anatomy and you can see from the crisscross design created by the angled position of our muscles that we were designed to control and create rotation.

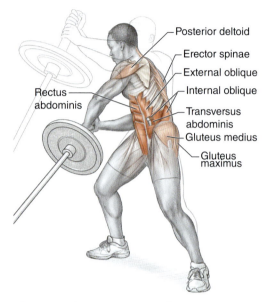

Figure 1.12   Some muscles may run vertically or horizontally, but many are aligned at angles that help us both control and create rotation.

This means we need to train the body to both resist and generate rotational forces. The concept of core stiffness discussed above is well known as an essential precursor to stability and efficient transfer of forces, not to mention injury prevention (Santana et al. 2015).

This bracing style of core training, also known as anti-rotation, is the best place to start when it comes to integrating more of the transverse plane, but we can't stop there. Every split-stance and unilateral exercise included in this book serves as a prime choice for challenging stiffness as the body must resist the rotational nature of the landmine with more traditional strength moves. The result is improved force transfer ability in what are known as the anterior and posterior slings of the body (see figure 1.12).

These slings are the synergistic groups of muscles and connective tissue on the front side (external obliques and opposite side adductors) and back side (lats and opposite side glutes) of the body that work together to transfer and control forces through the pelvis. These same muscles are also part of another concept known as the serape effect (see sidebar), often referred to as the X-factor, which further highlights the relationship between your shoulder and opposite hip in generating forces. Both concepts give us good reason to train with more split-stance and single-limb exercises like the ones discussed above to effectively train the control component of the transverse plane.

SERAPE EFFECT EXPLAINED

The serape effect describes the interaction of the obliques, serratus anterior, and rhomboids to transmit and stabilize rotational forces in the torso. This plays a vital role in rapid movements like sprinting, throwing, and striking, but it is also present in everyday activities like walking and stair climbing. This mechanism was named after the colorful woolen shawl worn in Mexico that is worn around the neck and tucked into the beltline in a fashion that resembles our crisscross muscular design. When the hips and shoulders rotate in opposite directions, it places these connected muscles under a prestretch (see figure 1.13). This prestretch is crucial in producing power and acceleration when the muscles contract. These muscles are designed to both generate and transmit forces and should be trained to both resist and create rotation between the hips and torso. This presents the potential for improved performance for explosive and rotational athletes, but it also plays a vital role in increasing midline stability for the everyday exerciser. These muscles also work together to increase core stability around the torso. When engaged together isometrically, they can help to stabilize the pelvis and minimize unwanted movement in an exercise.

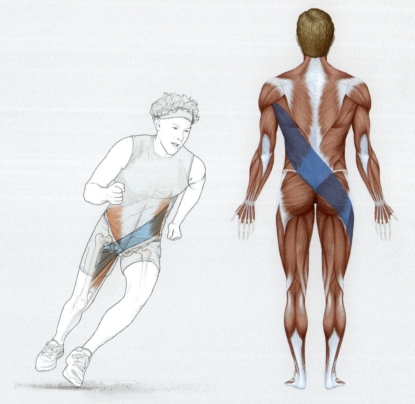

Figure 1.13   The synergistic muscular systems that help to transfer forces with most rotational and athletic movements.

The ability to generate stiffness in the core plays a vital role in performance and power transfer, but the idea of creating a prestretch in these slings of the body means that we also need to train them with rotation. Movement and rotation of the spine itself (bringing opposite hip and shoulder together) is essential in real-life power generation and should be safely trained.

The landmine allows for very simple to advanced progressions with a controlled and somewhat fixed bar path. This allows for users to quickly transition from focused rotation of the spine to training integrated rotation of the hips and core with zero change in setup or equipment.

Alternative Power Training

The benefits of power training and ballistic movements are well documented, but every exercise comes with a risk-to-reward ratio. Barbell Olympic lifts like the clean and snatch are great training tools for improving the rate of force production and athleticism and have long been considered the gold standard for improving power production. Unfortunately these movements require a great amount of skill and may present greater risk of injury due to common limitations in catching a barbell in the front rack or overhead position.

These types of lifts demand a level of wrist mobility and an overhead shoulder position (already mentioned) that most don't have, and they are also highly skilled exercises that take a significant time investment to master. For some, the investment may be warranted, but for many gym goers and recreational athletes, there are safer alternatives that are also easier to learn.

Unlike ballistic movements and power training with a traditional barbell or dumbbell, the landmine also has a fixed stopping point that almost serves as an additional point of contact and can be easier to control. Because of the landmine's single-end design and lateral stability demands, it's worth noting though that the overall loading potential may not be as high as other power alternatives.

However, the design of the landmine allows for a shorter learning curve with movements like the snatch or split jerk because they don't require the same catching positions that can make traditional Olympic lifts a challenge for the wrists and shoulders.

Versatility and Efficiency

The landmine is also known as "the corner gym" because of its versatility and efficiency as a training tool. If you're relatively new to the landmine, you will see from the exercises and programs in this book just how much high-quality work you can get done with a singular tool in a small space. For those who don't have hours to spend in the gym, this means less time wasted transitioning from one exercise setup to the next or waiting for a certain machine to become available. The result is more time for training and making gains.

The minimalist setup and design of the landmine also make it a great tool for home gyms, teams that may have multiple athletes training together, or environments where you may not have access to a ton of weight or equipment. Most moves demand a high level of stabilization throughout the entire kinetic chain—meaning that a bar and just a few plates is all you need to perform and intelligently progress exercises for the entire body.

Enhanced Grip Strength

Grip strength has long been tied to mortality and is one of the greatest predictors of functional capacity and mortality as we age. Although poor grip strength can be a limiting factor in some landmine exercises, it may also be your secret weapon for making improvements. The barbell end is thicker than most dumbbells and equipment, helping to explain its popularity in tactical training and combat sports.

The thicker diameter of the end of the barbell demands more from the muscles of the hand and forearm compared to the thinner grips of standard barbells and dumbbells. This increase in diameter forces users to engage their grip more intensively, strengthening the muscles involved and improving overall grip strength and endurance.

Additionally, the nature of landmine exercises—which often require dynamic, multidirectional movements—further intensifies the grip challenge. As exercisers perform movements such as presses, rows, or rotations, they must maintain a firm grip throughout the exercise's range, challenging their grip from all angles. This constant engagement not only builds strength but also mimics real-world activities where a strong, enduring grip is essential in picking up odd or large objects.

Incorporating landmine exercises into a training regimen offers practical benefits beyond typical strength gains. The grip-enhancing properties can improve performance in other lifts and daily activities, making landmine training a valuable component for athletes and fitness enthusiasts alike looking to develop a more robust and functional grip.

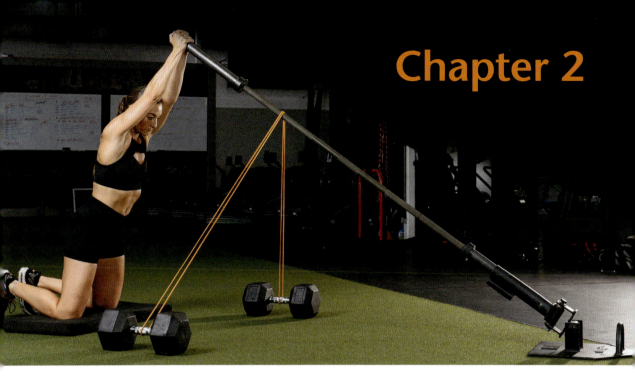

Chapter 2

SETUP, ATTACHMENTS, AND SAFETY

The appropriate setup for your landmine exercises will not only affect the effectiveness of your training but also your overall safety. In general, the landmine is an extremely safe training tool, and common risks that are associated with strength training can be easily mitigated with the proper setup. As with any exercise program, consultation with a healthcare provider is recommended, especially for those who have had muscle or joint injuries.

Follow the steps and suggestions in this chapter to make sure the risk-to-reward ratio remains in your favor as you explore all that the landmine has to offer.

COMMON LANDMINE SETUPS

Since the introduction of the Sorinex home base, many other landmine anchors have come on the market. This section covers a few of the most common setups, including the benefits and drawbacks of each based on the type of training and exercises you're looking to perform (see table 2.1).

Table 2.1 Landmine Setup Comparison

Type of setup	Ease of setup	Adjustable anchor height	Portable	Sturdiness (heavy or explosive moves)	Versatility
Rack attached	+	+	-	+	+
Home base	+	-	+	+	+
Plate insert	-	-	+	-	+
Slug-style cap	+	-	+	-	+

Rack Attached

If properly installed, especially to a strength training rack that is bolted to the ground, rack-attached landmines are the sturdiest of all the options for angled barbell training. Most attachments, such as the one in figure 2.1, will allow for mostly free movement because of the dual-pivot points but prevent shifting of the landmine during exercise regardless of the speed of movement or weight involved.

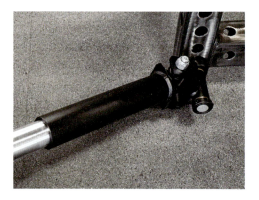

Figure 2.1 Rack-attached landmine.

Similar options are available that may be bolted to the ground or wall, and the benefits are the same as long as they are appropriately anchored.

Best For

- *Heavier strength exercises or explosive training movements.* The fixed position on the rack ensures that the landmine anchor does not slide on the ground due to heavy loading on one end or rapid movement of the bar.
- *Building efficient training stations for easy transition or multiple users.* This setup has become increasingly popular in group settings because of the ability to get a lot of training done with a minimal footprint.

- *Anyone who wants the possibility of varying the anchor height relative to the ground (i.e., higher anchor positions).* The exercises in this book are limited to anchor points closer to ground level, but the ability to alter the anchor height can open up additional exercise options.

Limitations

- *Requires additional equipment.* A rack-attached anchor requires a strength training rack of some kind as well as a commitment to bolting the attachment to the ground or wall.
- *Less mobile.* This anchor style means committing to the best placement for your landmine and making sure you have adequate space in front of and to the side of your rack to perform the desired exercises.

Home Base

Home base–style attachments are a sturdy but relatively mobile option for angled barbell training, with the name reflecting its similarity in shape to the home base plate used in baseball (see figure 2.2).

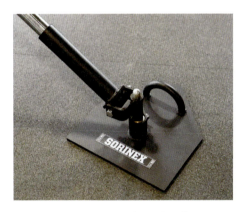

Figure 2.2 Home base landmine.

Best For

- *Nearly all landmine training for most users.* The landmine base itself is heavy enough and has enough surface-area contact with the floor so that it (generally) won't shift during training.
- *Freedom and flexibility in your position.* The home base can easily fit in a corner position or be moved around the room to accommodate training needs for the day. It is a great option for locomotive exercises that require a lot of lateral space on all sides of the landmine.

Limitations

- *Weight of the home base.* For smaller users, the home base can be relatively heavy. It may not be as easy to move around and store out of the way as some of the options that follow.
- *Potential for shifting.* As you start to work with heavier weights or place the home base on surfaces other than rubber gym flooring, the potential for shifting or sliding during an exercise increases.

Plate Insert and Drop-In

Plate insert and drop-in attachments offer creative ways of making use of already-available equipment by using the weight plates themselves as an anchor point that can be placed anywhere in the gym (see figure 2.3).

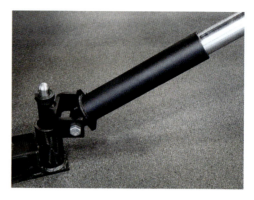

Figure 2.3   Plate insert or drop-in landmine.

Best For

- *Minimal investment to create a sturdy landmine training base.* Most of these attachments are relatively inexpensive in comparison to rack attachments and home base units. Just stack a few plates (preferably 45-pound [20 kg] bumper plates), drop it in, and go.
- *Flexibility and storage.* These attachments offer you the freedom to move your anchor point and then store everything out of the way when not in use.
- *Unrestricted motion in all directions.* Rack-mounted and even home base units may have blind spots that can prevent you from easily transitioning and continuing to use the equipment. Drop-in plate attachments enable you to maintain a relatively sturdy base while working in all directions around the plates.

Limitations

- *Can be cumbersome.* Setting up the plates themselves is easy but it can become cumbersome when setting up multiple plates if all the equipment is not conveniently located. Also, it is easier to use bumper plates than conventional weight plates due to their width.
- *Potential for shifting.* These types of attachments have the same potential for shifting as the home base setup when used with much heavier and more explosive training methods. They work best on rubber gym flooring or with plates wedged against a wall.

Slug-Style Cap

As the easiest grab-and-go anchor setup, slug-style barbell caps are simple in regard to getting started with angled barbell training but are more limited in use compared to some of the setups described earlier (see figure 2.4).

Best For

- *Minimal investment.* The slug-style cap requires minimal investment to perform landmine exercises while protecting your barbells, floors, and walls.

- *Placement against fixed surfaces.* Think of it as an upgrade over shoving your barbell into a corner.

- *Flexibility in placement and storage.* The Barbell Bomb pictured weighs next to nothing but is grippy enough to provide a relatively stable anchor point even in open floor spaces.

- *Versatility.* It can double as a handle on the working side as well.

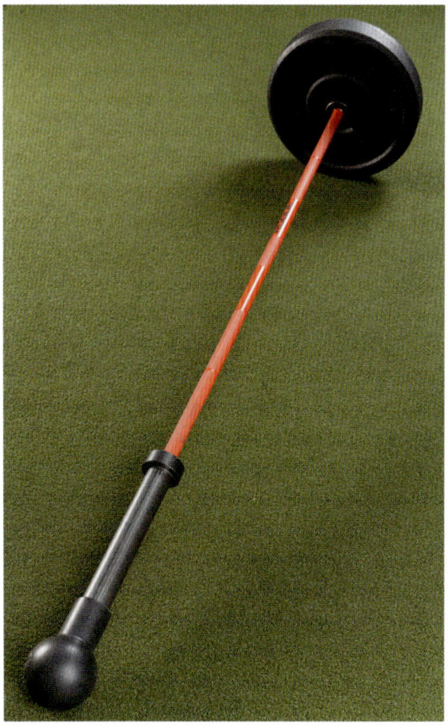

Limitations

- *Risk of movement.* It presents a greater risk of moving with heavier loading and power training, which can be overcome by ensuring they are placed on nonslip surfaces or against a fixed object.

- *Tipping hazard.* The potential for tipping hazards can arise with some movements, such as T-bar rows, if the leverage doesn't keep the anchor end wedged into a wall or on the ground.

Figure 2.4 Slug-style barbell cap.

ADVANCED SETUPS

Most of the exercises and programs listed in this book require simple setups, but there are a handful of slightly more involved setups that may make your training with the landmine more effective and efficient.

Elevated Starting Position

As your weight increases with the landmine in relation to your overall strength, one of the challenges can be the strength and position needed to lift the landmine from the floor. Although lifting the landmine has functional benefits, sometimes you may want to conserve energy or decrease the risk of injury during the start and end portions of your exercises. An elevated starting position may be used with vertical-pressing variations and squatting.

The two examples of "racked" setups in figure 2.5 can make it easier on your back when you are pushing with strength and intensity. These setups may also make it easier to add on and take off weight plates. Anyone who has trained with the landmine before knows how challenging it can be to put on and remove plates from the ground, so this setup can serve as a great solution, saving your strength and power for the exercises you're performing rather than when getting into the start position.

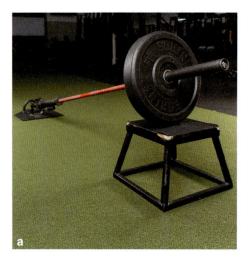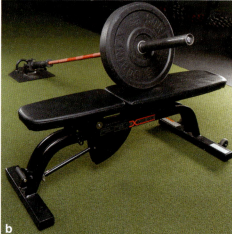

Figure 2.5   Using an elevated setup can increase training efficiency and challenges with getting heavy loads up from the floor.

SAFETY NOTE

This setup is best performed with a fixed rack- or wall-attached landmine because it creates a "lifting" effect on the anchored end of the barbell during the resting position with heavy loads. This can also be performed with the home base setup, but additional weights should be placed on top of the home base platform if more than 45 pounds (20 kg) are being added to the bar.

Accommodating Resistance (Adding Bands)

Accommodating resistance is a well-established method of training acceleration and power and can be a great way to amplify your landmine training. This training strategy is most commonly done with bands and chains to improve explosiveness, but we find bands to be more applicable to a wider variety of landmine exercises.

The following setups in figure 2.6 and 2.7 may be the best fit for the exercises in the power training section of this book. They can also offer a great progression of intensity and resistance for hypertrophy programs if done with controlled rather than explosive tempos. This may work well for those who enjoy the arc path of the landmine but don't want to lose tension or intensity while traveling up the arc of an exercise into a more vertical position.

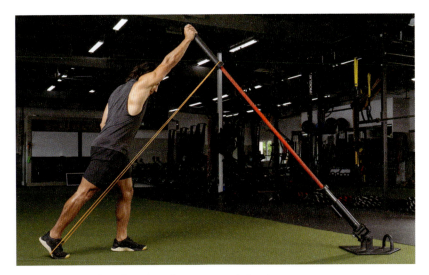

Figure 2.6   Band-resisted, staggered single-arm press.

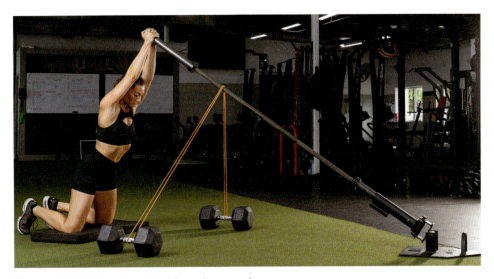

Figure 2.7   Band-resisted kneeling push press.

BEST ATTACHMENTS

Grip challenges and orientation have also been driving innovations in landmine attachments. Although none of these attachments are necessary to effectively train with the landmine, they may open up additional training exercises and options that are not within the scope of this book. This section is not meant to be an exhaustive list of all of the attachments and tools available for landmine training, but rather an overview of some of the most versatile and common landmine accessories.

Sleeve handles like the one pictured in figure 2.8 offer a smaller circumference grip for landmine exercises, which could allow for greater loading when grip is a limiting factor, such as with landmine rows. Exercisers who experience wrist discomfort with single-arm pressing or just smaller users with smaller hands may also benefit from the narrower grip. Distancing the grip farther from larger plates may also make some exercises more comfortable.

The Sorinex Griff handle (see figure 2.9) was built to solve the challenge that can occur when pressing the landmine with both hands. The bare landmine requires a slight amount of internal rotation for the shoulder; this handle more vertically aligns the forearms and allows for even better ergonomics when pressing heavier loads overhead. Most users will also find this grip relatively comfortable for heavy front loading, such as with the landmine goblet squat.

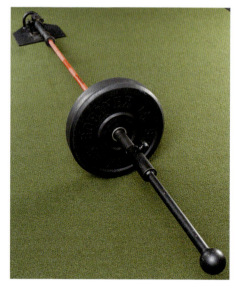

Figure 2.8 Sleeve handle.

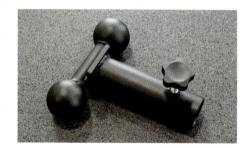

Figure 2.9 Landmine Griff handle.

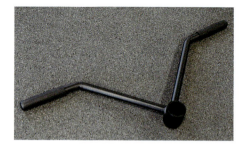

Figure 2.10 T-bar handle.

The slug-style caps pictured in the anchor options earlier in the chapter can also serve as a great handle attachment on the user end of the barbell. This may not only be a much more comfortable option for two-hand cradle exercises such as the goblet squat or thruster, but it can also be a great option for rotational core exercises such as rainbows.

The T-bar handle, if available, is a much better option for the T-bar row than the towel option demonstrated in the exercise section of this book. The T-bar handle (figure 2.10) allows for greater loading and also can serve as an alternative hand setup for exercises such as the overhead landmine row and core ticktocks.

LANDMINE SAFETY

Landmine training exercises as a whole are a safe method of strength training, but as with all weight lifting, there are some important things to keep in mind to minimize your risk of getting sidelined with unnecessary injury.

The most important thing is to ensure that your landmine anchor is secure and appropriate for the training you intend to do. Limitations were provided earlier in the chapter for some of the more common setups; these should be considered before picking up and using the landmine. Ensure that there is no risk of the ground side of the landmine sliding or shifting during exercises and that you have adequate space in all directions.

This means checking to ensure that any rack- or wall-attached landmines are properly secured and safe before use and testing that the home base–, drop-in–, and slug-style setups aren't going to move on you during the exercise.

The Pick-Up

Safety and great technique start with how you pick a weight up off the floor. The body was meant to be strong in a wide variety of positions, but it's in most users' self-interest to protect their back and be conscious of body position when picking up and setting down the landmine.

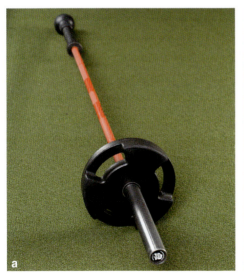 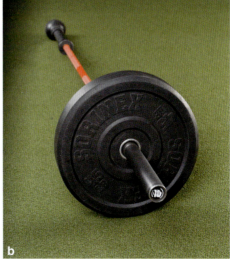

Figure 2.11   The height difference when using *(a)* traditional weight plates versus *(b)* larger bumper plates.

The unloaded landmine sits on the floor, so, when possible, use training plates or bumper plates like those pictured in figure 2.11 to bring it up to a height that is easier to lift to your starting position.

Also, refer to the examples and images of elevated starting positions presented earlier in the chapter for more efficient ways to set up the bar for heavier squatting and overhead-pressing exercises.

Start Light

If you're new to landmine training and some of the exercises included in this book, you should start with lighter weights and slower tempos. The stability demands of landmine training may be far greater than some of the traditional strength training exercises you have done in the past, so being conservative on overall loads will ensure that you perform the exercises with the correct technique.

This will help prevent injury and allow your neurological system to adapt, as well as set you up for far greater landmine gains in the months to come.

Landmine training is for everyone, but the weight of the bar can be a barrier for some. A standard barbell (45 pounds [20 kg]) may be too heavy for overhead and core movements. A more appropriate starting point for many exercisers would be to use a lighter training bar that weighs closer to 15 pounds (7 kg).

Get a Grip

Gripping the landmine presents some unique challenges based on the fact that a majority of exercises require holding the end of the barbell, which is much thicker than most exercise grips.

Although there are almost unlimited ways to grip and hold the landmine, the following three grips will cover almost all of your bases for the vast majority of landmine exercises.

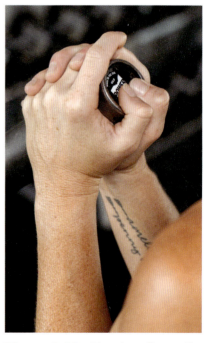

Two-Hand Cradle

Wedge the palms together at the very edge of the loading end of the landmine and make sure to interlace the fingers, if possible (figure 2.12). This is the most secure way to perform front-loaded lower body movements as well as any two-handed pressing variations. Avoid using one hand above or below the other as it may create uneven stress on the shoulders.

Figure 2.12 Two-handle cradle grip.

One-Arm Pressing

Although you may alter your hand position closer to or further away from the end of the barbell to impact torque or the perceived weight of the bar, you're generally best off holding at the far end for most exercises. The most important element here is for you to keep a stiff wrist like you would when throwing a punch so that the wrist is strong and stable. It will also help to start one-arm racked or pressing exercises with the forearm perpendicular to the barbell. Figure 2.13 shows the thumb at the end of the barbell instead of wrapped around because it tends to be most comfortable on the thumb; however, both positions are acceptable.

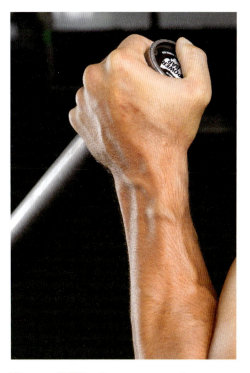

Figure 2.13   One-arm pressing grip.

One-Arm Pulling

This grip can be used with upper body pulling exercises as well as the holding position for single arm–held lower body exercises such as the single-leg Romanian deadlift (RDL). Placing the thumb around the end of the barbell (see figure 2.14) instead of wrapping it around the barbell shaft tends to offer a stronger grip for most exercisers and will generally allow for heavier lifting. If you are gripping the narrow portion of the bar for pulling exercises, then we suggest fully wrapping the hand around the barbell.

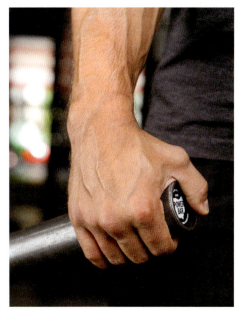

Figure 2.14   One-arm pulling grip.

BASE OF SUPPORT

One of the most common ways to progress an exercise is to adjust the base of support. Varying the foot position can alter muscular recruitment throughout the body and offers a simple way to customize exercise difficulty. Landmine training offers many options to progress from the most fundamental setups to very complicated and sport-specific options. Strength training demands generally require stable configurations with a minimum of one point of contact on the ground and optimally two for the most stable standing option. However, due to the lateral capabilities of the landmine, more performance-based stances are possible, allowing you to shift between points of contact and even leave points of contact.

These stances can be broken down into three categories: bilateral, which involves two points of contact throughout the entirety of the motion; transitional, which shifts between two points of contact and one point of contact through movement; and unilateral, which involves only one point of contact throughout the entirety of the motion.

Bilateral

- The two contact points can be broken down in many ways, from shoulder width apart to staggered and split-squat stances. The bilateral stance allows the lifter to shift their stability in a different direction (see figure 2.15).

- Staggered-stance exercises place greater stability demands on the muscles that control rotation and lateral motion because the load tends to be slightly off center.

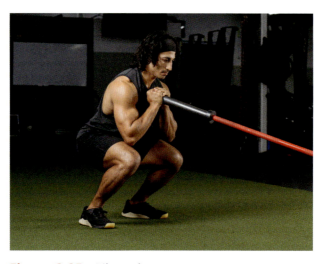

Figure 2.15   Bilateral stance.

Transitional

- This stance is most commonly seen with lunging (figure 2.16), shifting weight from two points of contact to one (or vice versa). This presents a greater balance and stability challenge because you are forced to control the momentum of the bar and restabilize your body and position with every step.

Unilateral

- Training with a single point of contact (figure 2.17) can increase the demand on the foot/ankle complex as well as the stabilization muscles in the hip.

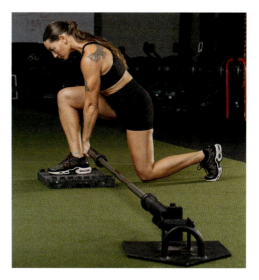

Figure 2.16   Transitional stance.

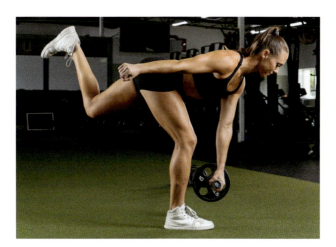

Figure 2.17   Unilateral stance.

This variety of base combinations enables exercisers to train with the landmine during all phases of their training journey. Although some stances are more advanced, stance orientation can amplify stability demands in combination with the existing requirements of the modality.

BETTER BAR PATH

A unique feature of landmine training is the path of the bar. Resistance training is all about placing force across muscles, and the direction in which the force is being applied (also known as a force vector) can have a big impact on the muscles that end up being used. Most free-weight activities exert a force directly downward due to gravitational pull. You may be able to place your body in various positions, but no matter what you do the free weight will only work vertically. While landmine training uses the same downward gravitational pull as free weights, the structure of the landmine is more complex. You can compare it to the ball-and-socket joints in the body. Like the shoulder and hip, the landmine has a fixed base and a lever that is mobile in a multidirectional capacity around the joint axis. With landmine movement, the fixed end of the barbell forces the weight to move in a semicircular path. As with the shoulder and hip joints in the body, the landmine offers the potential to create force in different directions, such as horizontally. The circular path of the bar can be advantageous for exercises like squats and presses because it may offer a more joint-friendly bar path.

Pressing patterns, specifically overhead pressing, can be challenging for exercisers due to the mobility requirements to get the weight directly overhead. Landmine pressing can be a joint-friendly option for people who cannot achieve full overhead mobility. Because the bar travels at an angled path, participants can press more forward than commonly seen in overhead pressing (similar to a high-incline press). For squatting, the bar path allows for a more angled body position, which more tightly correlates to certain athletic positions, as well as hack squatting options seen in gyms.

Although the barbell has been a reliable tool for power development, the angular path of the landmine provides an opportunity to work in changes in level and rotation. Moving weight from lower positions near the ground to overhead in one coordinated motion requires force transfer across the entire body, similar to many sports situations. From a rotational perspective, these types of movements can be accomplished in a more fluid, controlled, and explosive fashion than with other pieces of equipment, such as dumbbells or cable machines.

Mastering the proper setup, attachments, and safety considerations for landmine training will help you lay the foundation for success in the exercises to come. With the knowledge of how to safely and efficiently anchor your equipment, you can now explore the versatility that landmine training offers. The following chapters will dive into specific movements and techniques that harness the unique benefits of the landmine, enabling you to build strength, stability, and power in ways that traditional weightlifting methods may not.

As they say, "This is where the magic happens."

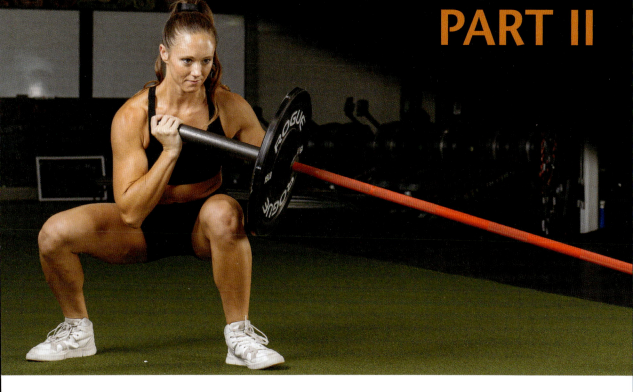

PART II

LANDMINE EXERCISES

In chapters 3 through 6, the landmine exercises are presented in order of difficulty and complexity within each chapter. Each exercise can be made more challenging with heavier loads, but the order in which they are presented should serve as a guide for your progression. Aim to master the exercises presented earlier in each chapter before jumping to the more challenging ones at the end. Keep in mind that although we tried to showcase as many variations as we could, the landmine is a versatile tool with almost infinite variations in stance and loading positions. We weren't able to include every possible landmine exercise, but the chapters that follow include the most effective landmine exercises for elevating your training.

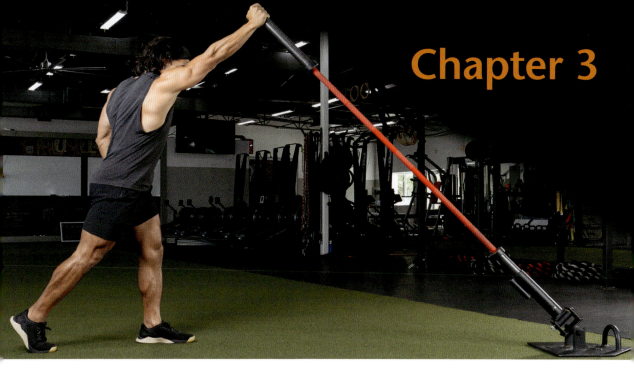

Chapter 3

UPPER BODY EXERCISES

This chapter includes landmine exercises geared toward building muscle, strength, and power in the upper body. The exercises are presented in push, pull, and accessory exercise categories throughout the chapter, with the majority of pushing and pulling upper body exercises being compound movements. Compound movements are preferred because they engage multiple muscle groups simultaneously, enhancing overall functional strength and improving coordination. As a training tool, you will find the landmine to be more beneficial in training compound versus isolation exercises.

Most of the exercises throughout this chapter are scalable for nearly any training level, but there is some skill associated with any new training tool. As a rough guide, the exercises in each section are presented in order of difficulty. Movements that require more coordination or balance will come after more stable exercises that are easier to execute. This doesn't make any of the exercises better than the others, but you would be best served to master the earlier moves in each section before jumping into those that require more skill and experience.

UPPER PUSHING EXERCISES

STANDING TWO-ARM LANDMINE PRESS

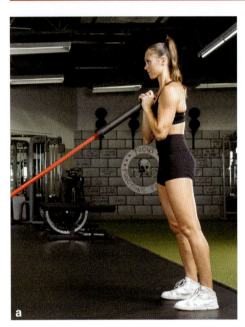
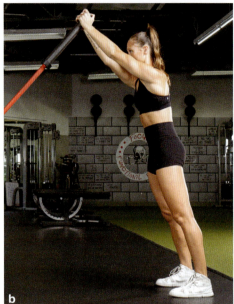

Muscles Targeted

This exercise targets the shoulders, triceps, and upper chest.

Starting Position

Stand facing the bar with the feet slightly wider than hip width and hands securely cradling the far end of the barbell with fingers interlaced. Body should be fully locked out with a very slight shift forward into the bar. Elbows should be tight to the ribs and hands right against the sternum (a).

Coaching Cues

• Brace the core and squeeze the quads to prevent unwanted movement in the torso.

• Press the barbell up and away from your body until your arms are fully locked out (b).

• Emphasize an active squeeze of the chest at the top.

• Slowly lower the barbell back down to the starting position.

Modifications

The exercise as it is pictured has both vertical and horizontal components, making it similar to an incline press when you keep the body relatively upright and minimize changes in your body angle. However, if you wish to mimic more of a direct overhead press, then you can lean into the barbell as you press up (c) to provide more vertical work for the shoulders and triceps.

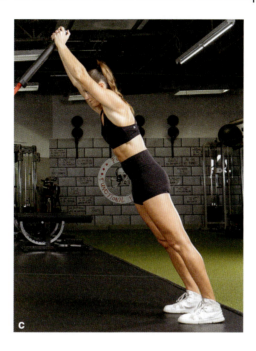

Tips

- Make sure to secure the barbell with a solid cradle grip (described in chapter 2) for safety and hold the elbows at approximately a 90-degree angle with the barbell at the bottom of each repetition.
- If you're looking to increase chest engagement, focus on squeezing the hands together on the bar throughout the exercise.

STANDING SHOULDER-TO-SHOULDER PRESS

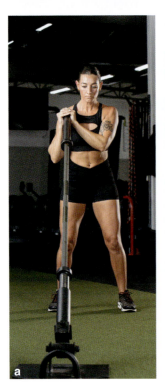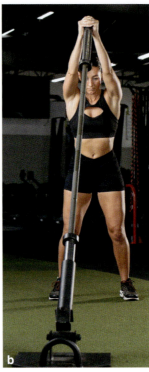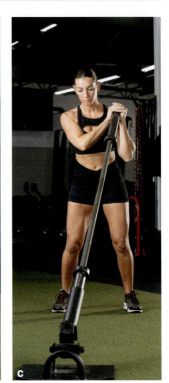

Muscles Targeted

This exercise targets the shoulders, triceps, and upper chest. It may also place a greater demand on the oblique muscles to resist lateral motion and rotation from the barbell.

Starting Position

Stand facing the bar, feet slightly wider than hip width, and body position locked out with a slight lean forward of your weight into the bar. Interlace your fingers and start with your hands placed in front of the right shoulder *(a)*.

Coaching Cues

- Brace the core and squeeze the quads to prevent unwanted movement in the torso.
- Press the barbell up and out away from the shoulder to a position centered in line with the body *(b)*.
- Slowly lower the barbell back down to the left shoulder *(c)* and repeat to the opposite side.

Modifications

Similar to the traditional two-arm press, the torso angle can also be altered in this exercise to create a more vertical overhead pressing motion. Although not pictured here (see kneeling two-arm press on page 48), this movement could also be performed from a full kneeling position for more direct overhead work as well as to increase the load on the upper body pushing muscles.

Tips

• Don't let the barbell drift outside of either shoulder position because it will take away from the upper body demand of the exercise and will instead place additional stress on the muscles of the core.

SINGLE-ARM PRESS

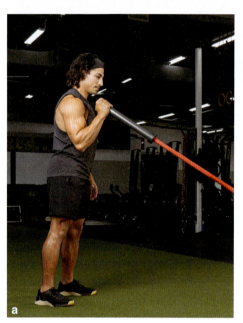 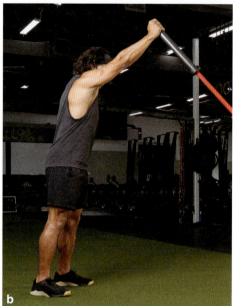

Muscles Targeted

This exercise primarily targets the shoulders and triceps, with some assistance from the chest. The offset load also increases demand on the rotational muscles of the core.

Starting Position

Stand facing the bar, feet slightly wider than hip width apart, and the landmine anchor in line with the right side of the body. Place the right hand securely around the end of the barbell in front of and just above the right shoulder. The wrist should be locked out and the forearm perpendicular to the bar *(a)* with the elbow close to the rib cage.

Coaching Cues

- Brace the core to minimize rotation or unwanted movement in the hips and core.
- Press the barbell straight up and away from your body relatively in line with the shoulder until your arm is fully locked out in line with the shoulder *(b)*.
- Slowly lower the barbell back down to the starting position.
- Perform the desired number of repetitions, then repeat on the left side.

Modifications

The position of the landmine relative to your stance can allow you to make this more of a stiff versus rotational press. The instruction above requires more torso stiffness, but placing the landmine anchor more to the center or even opposite side of the body allows for progression into more of a rotational pressing version of this exercise *(c)*. This version of the exercise can also be performed from the full kneeling position described later in this chapter.

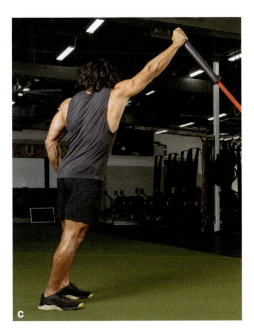

Tips

- Keep your weight shifted slightly more to the balls of the feet than the heels in this exercise. This will make it more natural for you to progress into rotational variations that require a more athletic stance.

STAGGERED SINGLE-ARM PRESS

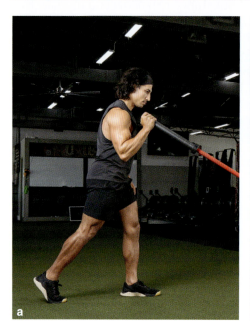
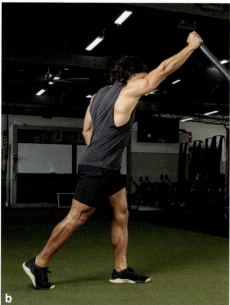

Muscles Targeted

This exercise primarily targets the shoulders and triceps, but the staggered stance turns this pressing exercise into a full body stability challenge as well.

Starting Position

Take a step back with the right foot and find a strong staggered stance while maintaining a soft bend in both the hips and knees of your left leg. Your right leg should be relatively straight with a strong foot position and heel off the ground. Align your right shoulder and hip with the anchor and hold the barbell in the right hand with a stiff wrist in front of the right shoulder *(a)*.

Coaching Cues

- Maintain a stiff back leg and slight forward lean and brace the core before initiating the exercise.
- Press the barbell straight up and away from your body until your arm is fully locked out in line with the shoulder *(b)*.
- Slowly lower the barbell back down to the starting position.
- Perform the desired number of repetitions, then repeat on the left side.

Modifications

This exercise is a foundational movement that can lead to a variety of upper body pushing and even full body power exercises. Aside from increasing the overall load, this exercise is a simple one to add accommodating resistance to by adding a resistance band to connect the barbell and the back foot *(c)*. You can also make this mimic more of a true overhead press by leaning your torso forward into the bar to press it directly overhead *(d)*.

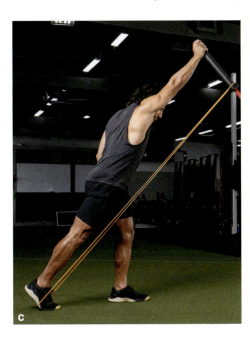
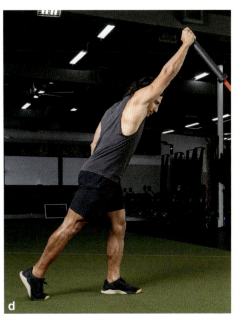

Tips

- The staggered stance introduces a higher level of stability and balance to the exercise, so don't take too narrow of a stance and minimize momentum with controlled lowering of the bar each rep.
- Use this as a pillar in your landmine training early on and it will open up better performance when doing more technical exercises down the road.

ROTATIONAL SINGLE-ARM PRESS

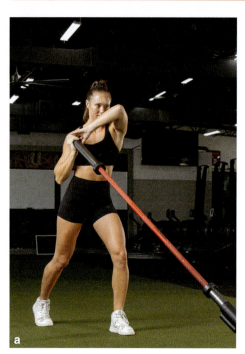
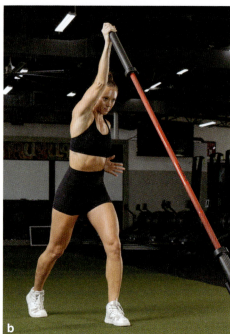

Muscles Targeted

This exercise primarily targets the shoulders and triceps, and the additional torso rotation brings in an element of power development from the lats and core.

Starting Position

Take a step back with the right foot and find a strong staggered stance while maintaining a soft bend in both the hips and knees of your left leg. Your right leg should be relatively straight with a strong foot position and heel off of the ground. Align your right shoulder and hip with the anchor and twist (coil) your torso toward the right leg to preload the core (a). Grip the barbell with the right hand and keep the right elbow tight to the rib cage with the left elbow pointed up in line with the anchor point.

Coaching Cues

- Maintain a stiff back leg and slight forward lean and rotate the torso enough to feel your lats engage on that side before the lift.
- Pull your left elbow down and away to the left side to rotate and explosively drive the barbell up with the right arm (b).
- Ensure that the rotation is occurring mostly above the hips in this movement.
- Slowly lower the barbell back down to the starting position.
- Perform the desired number of repetitions, then repeat on the left side.

Modifications

This exercise could be considered a progression of the staggered single-arm press because it adds some additional torso rotation and power to the pressing library of landmine exercises. The stance could also be switched for a slightly different training effect by placing the same leg forward on the side that is lifting instead of back. This will translate more into the step-through press found in the full body/hybrid moves found later in chapter 5.

Tips

- The concept of coiling the core may go against the technique stiffness that you are used to in training, but it can be great for training the athletic rotation we all use in daily life.

- Start light with the movement and focus on feeling the lats before initiating the exercise, then explode with the opposite elbow to take advantage of your body's rotational design.

- Over time as you add load and speed, this movement will begin to feel more natural.

KNEELING LANDMINE PRESS

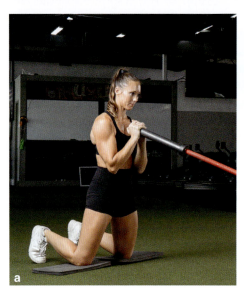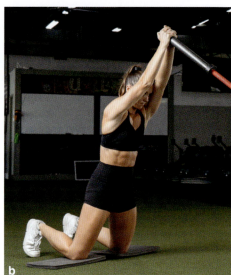

Muscles Targeted

This exercise targets the shoulders, triceps, and upper chest.

Starting Position

Assume a strong full kneeling position facing the end of the barbell by placing the knees directly below the hips, squeezing the glutes, and digging the toes into the ground. The body should be fully locked out with a very slight shift forward into the bar. Elbows should be tight to the ribs and hands right against the sternum (a).

Coaching Cues

- Brace the core and squeeze the glutes to keep the pelvis locked into place.
- Press the barbell up and away from your body until your arms are fully locked out (b).
- Emphasize an active squeeze of the chest at the top.
- Slowly lower the barbell back down to the starting position.

Modifications

The full kneeling position can also be used in the shoulder-to-shoulder (page 40) and single-arm press (page 42) exercises. The main difference will be the greater load presented in the kneeling position because of the more vertical path of the barbell toward the bottom of its arc.

Tips

- Keep in mind that any of the standing-pressing variations in this chapter will feel heavier in the kneeling stance position when using the same load because of the body's position relative to the landmine load and the bar path. Decrease the load used to accommodate the intensity.

- This is also a great exercise to take advantage of the elevated position landmine setup described in chapter 2, because heavier loads can be challenging to lift into position on your own when using kneeling and half-kneeling stances.

HALF-KNEELING SINGLE-ARM PRESS

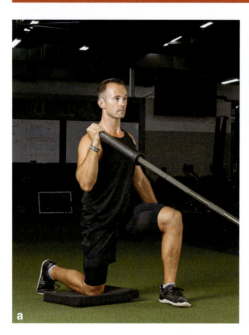
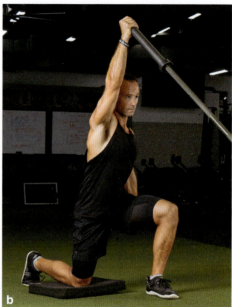

Muscles Targeted

This exercise primarily targets the shoulders and triceps; the half-kneeling position also demands a significant amount of hip and core stability.

Starting Position

Assume a half-kneeling position by placing the right knee directly underneath your hips with your back toe dug into the ground in line with the hip. Place your left foot directly in front of your left hip at approximately 90-degree angles for the hip and knee. Grip the barbell with the right hand directly in front of your right shoulder *(a)*.

Coaching Cues

- Dig your back toes into the ground and squeeze the glute of the kneeling leg to help lock the hips and core into place.
- Press the barbell straight up and away from your body until your arm is fully locked out in line with the shoulder *(b)*.
- Slowly lower the barbell back down to the starting position.
- Perform the desired number of repetitions, then repeat on the left side.

Modifications

This exercise will feel heavier relative to the same load than standing variations because of the increased level of torque from the barbell in a lower position. This may necessitate using a lighter training bar for smaller exercisers or self-assisting with the opposite hand, as needed.

Tips

- Keep digging the back toes into the ground for greater stability throughout; make sure your starting position allows you to have a slight forward lean of the torso.
- Place the hand at the far end of the landmine for optimal leverage and maintain a stiff wrist position.

HALF-KNEELING LATERAL PRESS

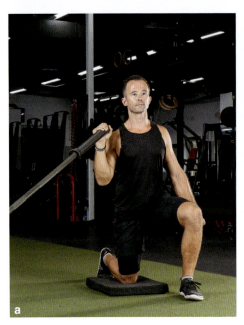
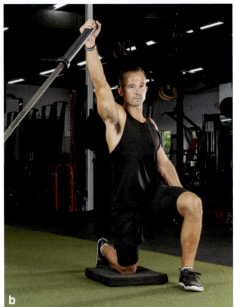

Muscles Targeted

This exercise targets the muscles of the shoulders and triceps.

Starting Position

Assume a strong half-kneeling position with your body faced approximately 45 degrees away from the landmine anchor point and your right toes dug into the ground. Grip the far end of the barbell with your right hand held just above the right shoulder, keeping your right arm tight against the rib cage *(a)*.

Coaching Cues

- Before lifting, make a fist with the left hand and brace the core to create some stiffness.
- Press the right arm up and away from the body into a locked-out position *(b)*.
- Slowly lower back down to the starting position.
- Perform the desired number of repetitions, then repeat on the left side.

Modifications

Based on your shoulder flexibility, you may angle your body slightly more or less than 45 degrees away from the landmine anchor point to create the ideal bar path for your shoulder. This exercise is also great to perform from a true lunge position with the back knee off the ground to add in some lower body isometrics *(c)*.

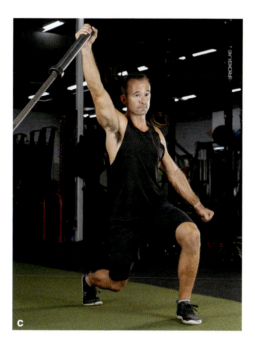

Tips

• This pressing variation will likely be much weaker compared to the standard single-arm press angle, so start with lighter loads to fine-tune your start position and pressing technique.

SEATED SINGLE-ARM PRESS

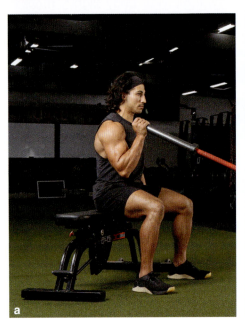
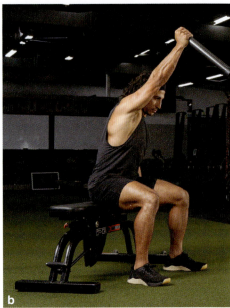

Muscles Targeted

This exercise primarily targets the shoulders and triceps, along with some assistance from the chest muscles.

Starting Position

Sit tall at the edge of a bench or box that allows for close to 90-degree angles at both the hips and knees. Feet should be kept planted on the ground about hip width apart and the torso held relatively upright. Hold the end of the barbell in the right hand. The right elbow should be tight to the ribs and the right hand stacked right above it (a).

Coaching Cues

- Brace the core and keep the left arm locked out with fist held tight to generate maximal body tension.
- Press the barbell up and away from your body until your right arm is fully locked out *(b)*.
- Emphasize an active lockout of the arm at the top and strong shoulder position.
- Slowly lower the barbell back down to the starting position.
- Perform the desired number of repetitions, then repeat on the left side.

Modifications

This same seated start position could also be used to perform two-arm (page 38) and shoulder-to-shoulder (page 40) pressing variations.

Tips

- Lifting the weight up into position and then sitting down can be awkward, so, if possible, take advantage of the elevated start position and setup described in chapter 2 for more efficient training with this pressing exercise.

ROLLOUT PUSH-UP

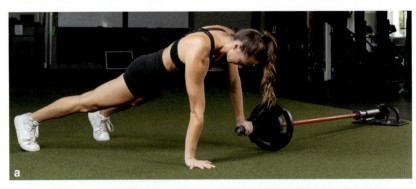

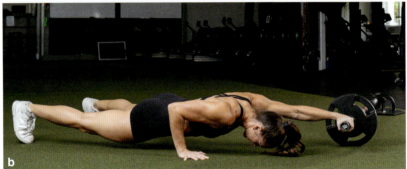

Muscles Targeted

This exercise targets the shoulders, triceps, and upper chest.

Starting Position

Position yourself on the floor perpendicular to the barbell on your hands and knees, hands planted directly below your shoulders and knees planted directly below your hips. Using your inside hand closest to the barbell, grab onto the end of the barbell. Walk your legs out behind you and lift the knees off the floor until you're in the push-up position, weight on your hands and toes *(a)*.

Coaching Cues

- Maintain a tall spine throughout the entirety of the movement.
- Squeeze your quads to maintain the hip position.
- Lower down into a push-up while the landmine arm rolls away and in front of you *(b)*.
- Imagine pushing the floor away from you with the grounded hand to return to the starting position and roll the barbell back in.
- Emphasize an active squeeze of the chest at the top.
- Perform the desired number of repetitions, then repeat on the other side.

Modifications

The most basic way to modify this exercise is to shorten the range of motion. Specifically, with the landmine-based hand, it may be easiest to place a plate on the floor in the path of the bar as far as you are comfortable moving. This forces the motion to be limited rather than navigating it on your own.

SINGLE-ARM Z-PRESS

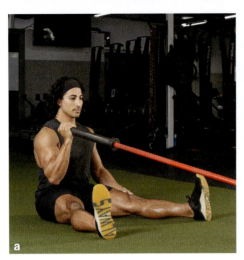
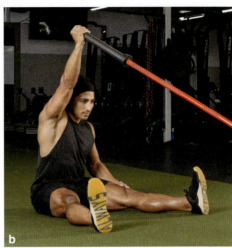

Muscles Targeted

This exercise targets the shoulders, triceps, and upper chest, while also increasing the stability demand of all muscles connecting to the pelvis.

Starting Position

Sit on the ground with legs spread approximately 45 degrees from parallel. Do your best to maintain a natural curvature of the spine. Place the end of the barbell in your right hand in line with the shoulder *(a)*.

Coaching Cues

- Maintain a strong tall torso position as you brace your core before pressing the weight.
- Press the barbell overhead until your right arm is fully locked out in line with the shoulder *(b)*.
- Maintain the body position and slowly lower the barbell back down to the starting position.
- Perform the desired number of repetitions, then repeat on the left side.

Modifications

This movement requires a high level of adductor and hamstring flexibility as well as pelvic stability. If the proper position cannot be maintained from the floor, the exercise can be modified by elevating the butt onto pads or a very small box. This movement could also be performed with two hands and would target muscles similar to the standing landmine press.

Tips

- This is not the pressing variation that you should try to hit a personal record with, but one that should be used to provide an additional challenge for the mobility and strength of the hips and pelvis.
- Start with lighter loads and stay focused on perfect position with this pressing exercise before increasing the load.

SINGLE-ARM FLOOR PRESS

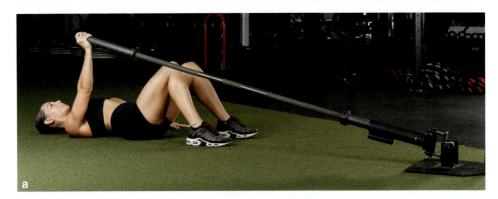

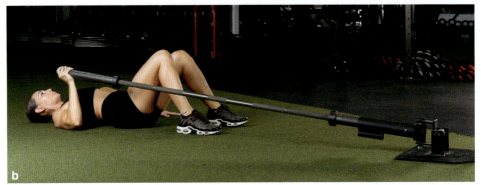

Muscles Targeted

This exercise targets the chest, shoulders, and triceps.

Starting Position

Lie parallel to the barbell on your back near the far end of the landmine with your head in line with the landmine anchor. Bend your knees so your feet are placed firmly on the ground just outside of hip width. Lift the barbell off the ground with both hands and then grip it firmly with your right hand locked out in line with the bottom of your chest *(a)*.

Coaching Cues

- Squeeze the left hand and brace the core to create tension before lowering the weight.
- Slowly lower the weight toward the ground by bending the right elbow to about a 40- to 60-degree angle in relationship to your body *(b)*.
- Stay engaged at the bottom and don't let the elbow crash down to the ground.
- Drive the weight back up into a locked-out and controlled position.
- Perform the desired number of repetitions, then switch to the left arm.

Modifications

This movement can also be performed from a bridge position with the hips off the floor *(c)* to increase the range of motion relative to the shoulder and change the pressing angle.

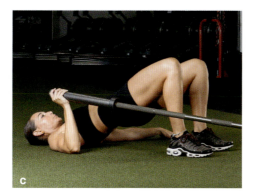

Tips

- Getting into your start position can be challenging with much heavier weights, so opt for a spotter to help you lift the landmine into position when handling heavier loads.
- You may also find that you need to shift slightly closer to or further away from the barbell once you are in your starting position to find your ideal bar path.

STANDING CHEST FLY

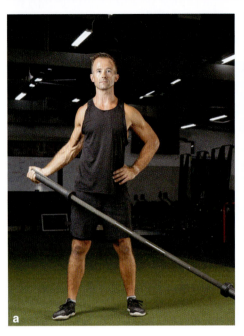
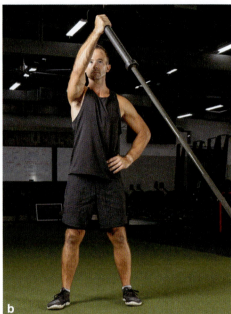

Muscles Targeted

This exercise targets the chest as well as the anterior shoulders.

Starting Position

Stand with feet slightly wider than hip width, angled 45 degrees away from the landmine anchor point. Grip the barbell at the far end of the collar with your right hand, positioned along your side and elbow slightly bent *(a)*.

Coaching Cues

- Place the left hand on your core to make sure you are braced before lifting.
- While maintaining a slight bend in the right elbow, raise the bar up and across the body toward your left side.
- Actively squeeze your chest at the top *(b)*.
- Maintain chest engagement and slowly lower back to the starting position.
- Perform the desired number of repetitions, then switch to the left arm.

Modifications

This exercise is relatively challenging for most people with even just the unweighted bar because of the long arm lever position. That being said, this one may be best to start with a lighter bar when possible to ensure adequate reps and appropriate technique.

Tips

• The angle of your body in relation to the landmine anchor will make a big impact on engaging the right muscles, so start with a 45-degree angle relative to the anchor point.

• Don't hesitate to tweak from there until you feel a significant amount of chest engagement, especially in the top half of the range of motion.

UPPER PULLING EXERCISES

TWO-HANDED LANDMINE ROW (PRISON ROW)

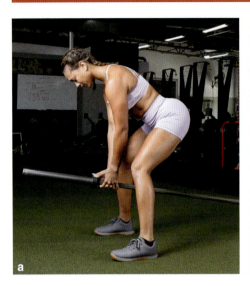
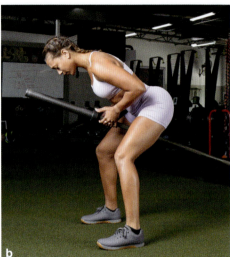

Muscles Targeted

This exercise engages most of the major muscles of the back, with an emphasis on the lats, rear deltoids, and biceps.

Starting Position

Assume a foot position slightly wider than your normal Romanian deadlift (RDL) or slightly wider than hip width and grip the barbell with a hand-over-hand or interlaced-finger position as close to the collar as your setup allows. Create a soft bend in the knees and maintain a neutral spine position as you hinge your hips to about 45 degrees *(a)*.

Coaching Cues

- Maintain core stiffness and a strong lower body position to minimize low back stress.
- Draw the elbows back and pull the barbell up as close to your body as possible *(b)*. Slowly lower back to the starting position.

Modifications

This exercise can build isometric strength in the lower back, but assume a higher torso angle if you find yourself unstable or feel pain in the low back. If you're looking for more range of motion in this position, add a towel *(c)*, or see the T-bar row variation.

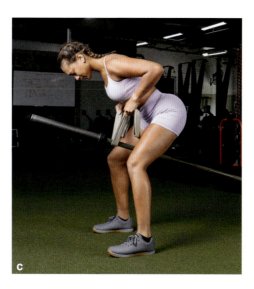

Tips

- Olympic-sized plates (larger diameter) are nice for most landmine exercises as you lift the weight off of the ground, but they can get in the way of the body during this exercise.
- If possible, use smaller 10-pound and 25-pound plates to minimize any interference from the plates.

VARIATION: T-BAR ROW

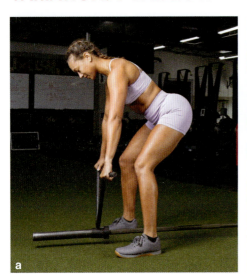 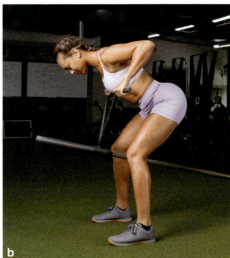

Muscles Targeted

This exercise engages most of the major muscles of the back with an emphasis on the lats, rear deltoids, and biceps.

Starting Position

Assume a foot position slightly wider than your normal RDL and grip each side of the T-bar handle on the barbell as close to the collar as you can. Create a soft bend in the knees and maintain a neutral spine position as you hinge your hips to around or slightly greater than 45 degrees *(a)*.

Coaching Cues

- Maintain core stiffness and a strong lower body position to minimize low back stress.
- Draw the elbows back and pull the weight until the hands are outside of the ribs and chest *(b)*.
- Slowly lower back to the starting position.

Modifications

This exercise can be great at building isometric strength in the lower back, but assume a higher torso angle if you find yourself unstable or in pain in the low back. The T-bar handle allows for a wider hand position and greater range of motion in comparison to the two-handed landmine row (prison row), but it can also easily be substituted with a triceps rope or towel *(c)*. The towel version is purposely grip intensive, so keep that in mind when selecting loads.

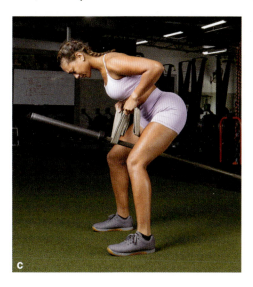

Tips

- Olympic-sized plates (larger diameter) are nice for most landmine exercises as you lift the weight off of the ground, but they can get in the way of the body during this exercise for shorter exercisers.
- If needed, use smaller 10-pound and 25-pound plates to minimize this issue or elevate the feet on blocks to adjust the range of motion and angles.

STAGGERED SINGLE-ARM ROW

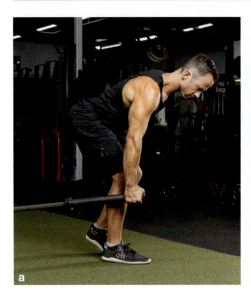 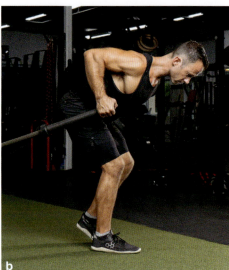

Muscles Targeted

This exercise targets the lats and biceps.

Starting Position

Standing at the very end of the barbell, grip the barbell collar with the right hand as close to the end as possible. Assume a staggered stance by placing the left foot just behind the right and keeping the left heel off the ground. Hinge the hips to about 45 degrees and place most of your weight onto the right leg *(a)*.

Coaching Cues

- Brace the core and drive the right foot hard into the ground to create stability in your starting position.
- Pull the right elbow back so the right hand travels up and back to the bottom of your rib cage and then squeeze the lats *(b)*.
- Slowly lower back to the starting position.
- Perform for the desired number of repetitions, then switch to the left arm.

Modifications

This exercise develops isometric hip and core stability, but you may need to make some small shifts in your stance to get into what feels like your power stance with this movement. This exercise can also be completed with identical coaching cues and setup from an even (versus staggered) stance. Grip may be a limiting factor for those with smaller hands or when using heavier weights, so this could be a great opportunity to use a handle attachment if available for a smaller grip diameter *(c)*.

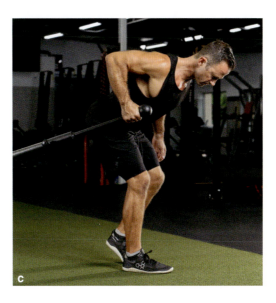

Tips

- For better grip during the exercise, maintain a hook grip (as pictured) by not wrapping the thumb around the collar of the bar.
- This will also help you maintain a focus on using the lats in this exercise and not rely too heavily on the biceps.

MEADOWS ROW

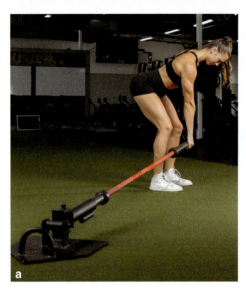 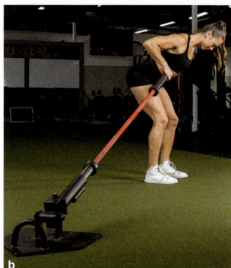

Muscles Targeted

This exercise targets the lats as well as the upper back muscles, biceps, and forearms.

Starting Position

Standing with an even hip-width stance perpendicular to the barbell, grip the far end of the collar with your right hand. Hinge your hips back so that your torso is in a strong position just above parallel with the ground. The very end of the barbell collar should sit just inside of your right foot when at the starting position (a).

Coaching Cues

- Press the feet firmly into the ground and brace the core to create core strength and stiffness before starting the movement.
- Pull the right elbow up and back so the right hand and barbell travel up to the bottom ribs (b).
- Slowly lower back to the starting position.
- Perform the desired number of repetitions, then repeat on the left side.

Modifications

The unsupported Meadows row described here is great for building positional core and hip strength, but it can also be done from a supported position *(c)*. The supported version allows for significantly heavier loading and focuses more on the muscles of the back without being limited by the core. To target the upper back more than the lats, you can pull the barbell toward the chest rather than the ribs and allow the elbow to travel further out away from the body.

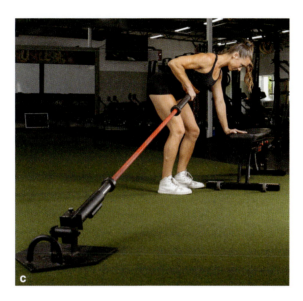

Tips

- Torso angle is just a suggestion here; those with much longer limbs may need to maintain a higher position to avoid low back strain, so find what feels best while maintaining proper form.
- Once you have built some solid strength and confidence here, the supported Meadows row can be a great pulling move with heavier weight, so use this one to build some serious strength.

VARIATION: STAGGERED MEADOWS ROW

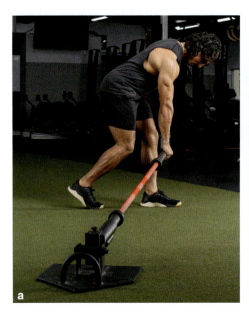 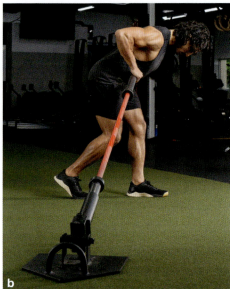

Muscles Targeted

This exercise targets the lats as well as the upper back muscles, biceps, and forearms.

Starting Position

Assume a staggered stance slightly smaller than your normal lunge position with the left leg forward perpendicular to the line of the barbell *(a)*. Grip the far end of the collar with your right hand. Hinge your hips back and slightly bend both knees so your torso is 45 degrees or less in relation to the ground. The very end of the barbell collar should sit just inside of your right hip when at the starting position.

Coaching Cues

- Brace the core and drive firmly through the left foot to create stability in the start position before lifting.
- Pull the right elbow up and back so the right hand and barbell travel up to the bottom ribs *(b)*.
- Slowly lower back to the starting position.
- Perform the desired number of repetitions, then repeat on the left side.

Modifications

The unsupported staggered Meadows row seen in the primary images is great for building positional hip and isometric glute strength, but it can also be done from a supported position *(c)*. The supported version will allow for significantly heavier loading, focus more on the muscles of the back, and engage the front side of the core with the opposing hand driving through a bench or box. If you don't have a box, then placing the nonworking elbow on your front thigh can also work well. To work more of the upper back than the lats, you can also pull the barbell more toward the chest than the ribs and allow the elbow to travel further out away from the body.

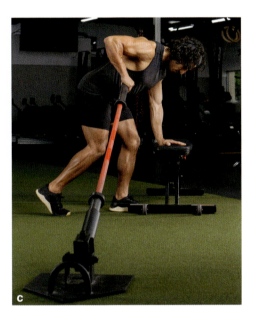

Tips

- Torso angle is just a suggestion here; those with much longer limbs may also need to maintain a higher position to avoid low back strain, so find what feels best while maintaining proper form.

SINGLE-LEG RDL ROW

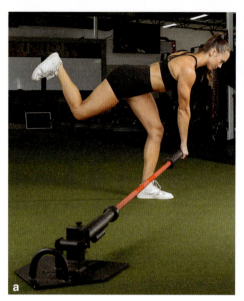
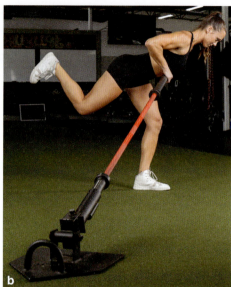

Muscles Targeted

This exercise targets the upper back and lats as well as a high level of hip and isometric core strength due to the single-leg position.

Starting Position

Grip the far end of the collar with your right hand held just inside of the left foot. Maintain a soft bend in the left knee and hinge at the left hip to bring your right leg off the ground behind you with your thigh as close to parallel with the ground as possible. Keep your back in a neutral position and hold your left hand out to the side for balance *(a)*.

Coaching Cues

- Squeeze the left fist and maintain solid glute engagement on the left leg to create a strong starting position.
- Pull the right elbow up and back so the right hand and barbell travel up to the bottom ribs *(b)*.
- Slowly lower back to the starting position.
- Perform the desired number of repetitions, then repeat on the left side.

Modifications

If it's a challenge to keep your balance, lightly place the left hand on a bench or box.

Tips

- This pulling variation is not going to be the place for personal lifting records, but more of a way to build hip and back strength. With this in mind, focus on controlled tempos and isometrics rather than on chasing strength.
- Make sure you have been simultaneously building posterior chain strength with landmine RDLs and standard rows before combining them with this exercise.

UPPER BODY ACCESSORY EXERCISES

UPRIGHT ROW

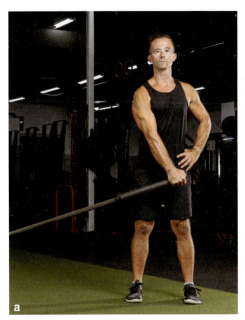 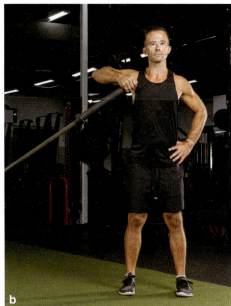

Muscles Targeted

This exercise targets the deltoids and traps along with a little bit of forearm work.

Starting Position

Stand with the feet hip width apart, torso relatively upright, and grip the barbell in the right hand. The end of the barbell should sit just inside of the left leg at the starting position (a).

Coaching Cues

- Maintain stiffness throughout the body and keep the right thumb on the end of the barbell instead of wrapped around.
- Drive the right elbow up and out away from the body so the right hand finishes in front of the right shoulder (b).
- Slowly lower back to the starting position.
- Perform the desired number of repetitions, then repeat on the left side.

(continued)

Upright Row *(continued)*

Modifications

This exercise targets the deltoids and traps, but the grip and weight of the bar may present as limitations for some. Alternative handle attachments may assist in making this exercise more manageable, and a lighter training bar may be best for smaller exercisers.

Tips

- Don't let the hand get higher than the elbow on this one in order to maintain good technique and minimize stress on the rotator cuff.
- Think about leading up and out with the elbow.

LATERAL RAISE

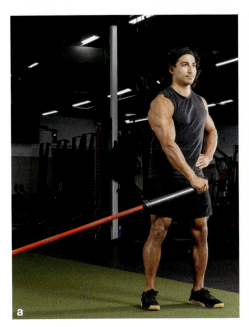 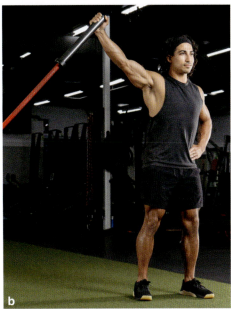

Muscles Targeted

This exercise targets the shoulder.

Starting Position

Stand with the feet hip width apart, torso upright, and grip the barbell in the right hand at the very end. Your body should be perpendicular to the bar, and the end of the barbell should sit just inside of the left leg at the starting position (a).

Coaching Cues

- Maintain stiffness throughout the body and a very slight bed in the right arm to avoid lockout.
- Bring the right hand up and out away from the body in an arced path with the barbell until it is in line with the body (b).
- Slowly lower back to the starting position.
- Perform the desired number of repetitions, then repeat on the left side.

Modifications

This exercise provides a unique path for the weight, but even unloaded is fairly heavy for most. If you can't normally lateral raise 20- to 25-pound dumbbells, opt for a lighter training bar to maintain proper technique.

Tips

- Don't let the bar get away from you at the top position.
- Make sure to stop just in line or short of being in line with the body.

CONCENTRATION CURL

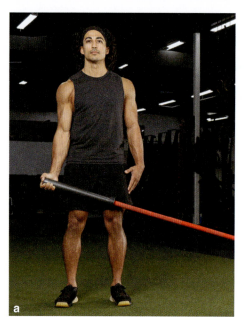
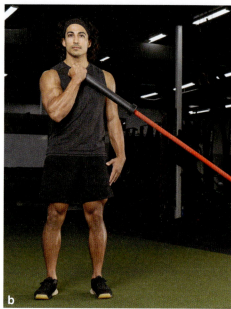

Muscles Targeted

This exercise targets the biceps.

Starting Position

Stand with the feet hip width apart, torso upright, and grip the barbell in the right hand with the palm facing up. Your body should be perpendicular to the bar and the upper right arm should be tight to the rib cage *(a)*.

Coaching Cues

- Maintain stiffness throughout the body and keep the right arm fixed tightly to the body.
- Curl the landmine up and slightly across the body to the top of the chest *(b)*.
- Slowly lower back to the starting position.
- Perform the desired number of repetitions, then repeat on the left side.

Modifications

The barbell alone here can be challenging to lift, so you may also opt for the mixed-grip curl (page 79) as a way to use your inside hand for assistance in reaching a certain rep range.

Tips

- Keep the thumb outside of the barbell (as pictured) rather than wrapped tightly around the bar to maximize biceps and minimize forearm fatigue.
- Use an extended handle attachment for this one, if needed; this may be especially helpful for smaller hand sizes.

MIXED-GRIP CURL

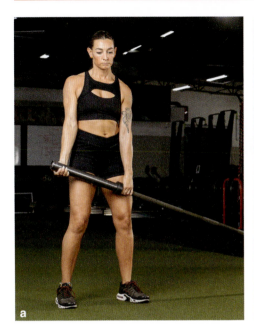
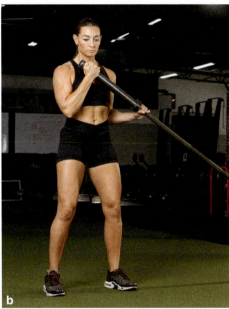

Muscles Targeted

This exercise targets the biceps and forearm muscles, specifically the brachio-radialis.

Starting Position

Stand with the feet hip distance apart, torso upright, and grip the barbell with both hands. The right hand should be palm-up at the bar end of the barbell and your left hand should grip the bar with an overhand grip just below the collar of the bar. Your body should be perpendicular to the bar and centered on the barbell collar (a).

Coaching Cues

• Maintain stiffness throughout the body, with the shoulders pulled back and down.

• Using both arms simultaneously, curl the barbell up and across the body until the right hand is positioned at the top of the chest (b).

• Slowly lower back to the starting position.

• Perform the desired number of repetitions, then repeat on the left side.

(continued)

Mixed-Grip Curl *(continued)*

Modifications

You can play with different hand positions to bias either arm during the exercise, but if experiencing any consistent elbow pain, start with fewer sets and load on this exercise to slowly build strength in the flexors and extensors of the forearm.

Tips

- This variation overloads the biceps in the outside arm by using a little assistance from the inside arm.
- Try using both arms on the way up and then just the outside arm on the way down for an eccentric overload challenge!

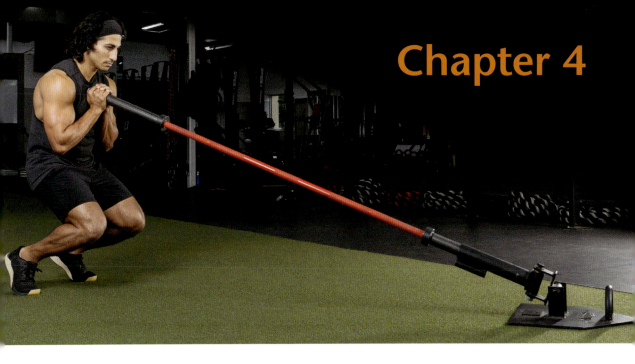

Chapter 4

LOWER BODY EXERCISES

This chapter includes landmine exercises geared toward building muscle, strength, and power in the muscles of the lower body. The landmine shines as a total body training tool, but this chapter on lower body exercises contains the greatest number of exercises and variations. The exercises are presented in squat, lunge, and hinge categories to help you organize your training. Categorizing exercises in this way is beneficial because it ensures a balanced and comprehensive approach to lower body development. It also helps you target different movement patterns, improving overall functional strength and reducing the risk of injury by promoting balanced muscle development and joint stability.

Much like the upper body exercises presented in chapter 3, the majority of movements presented in this chapter are compound exercises because the landmine as a tool is more limited when it comes to isolation work. The exercises in each category are listed in order of increasing skill level. Movements introduced earlier tend to be those that are easier to execute well with minimal coaching, whereas some of the later exercises require some skill and practice to get the most out of them.

SQUATTING EXERCISES

LANDMINE GOBLET SQUAT

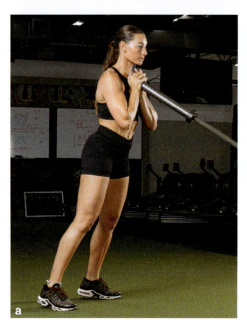
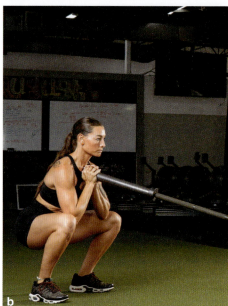

Muscles Targeted

This exercise could be considered full body because of the front-loaded demand on the core, but it primarily targets the quadriceps, upper back, and glutes.

Starting Position

Interlace your fingers to securely grip the far end of the landmine held tightly against the sternum. Place your feet slightly wider than hip width and assume a slight lean into the landmine. Weight should be shifted forward slightly into the balls of the feet *(a)*.

Coaching Cues

- Inhale and brace your core, holding the arms tight to the body.
- Simultaneously bend at the hips and knees, slowly dropping back and down into the bottom position, ideally with thighs parallel to the ground *(b)*.
- Keep the core braced, drive your feet through the ground, and exhale as you push back up to the starting position.

Modifications

Torso lean and foot placement can have a significant impact with this exercise, so, like most squatting movements, you should play with stances and positions to find the position you feel strongest in. There is no one-size-fits-all squatting stance, so hone in on where you feel strongest and can train the greatest range of motion. Once you find this position, you can also modify your torso lean to create more or less horizontal force production (see discussion in chapters 1 and 2 for potential benefits of this).

Tips

- Interlace your fingers and hold the wrists tight together against the chest to maintain a solid rack position.
- As the weights get heavier, lifting the landmine from the floor to the starting position can become challenging. We recommend using a spotter or elevated starting position when possible.

VARIATION: HEELS-ELEVATED SQUAT

Muscles Targeted

This exercise could be considered full body because of the front-loaded demand on the core, but it primarily targets the quadriceps, upper back, and glutes.

Starting Position

Interlace your fingers to securely grip the far end of the landmine held tightly against the sternum. Place your feet slightly wider than hip width and assume a slight lean into the landmine. Weight should be shifted forward slightly into the balls of the feet and the heels elevated onto plates (a) or wedges (b).

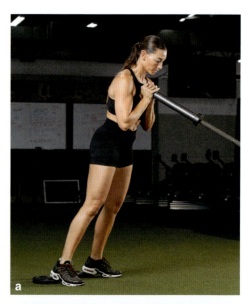

Coaching Cues

- Inhale and brace your core with arms held tight to the body.
- Simultaneously break at the hips and knees, slowly dropping back and down into the bottom position, ideally with thighs parallel to the ground (c).
- Keep core braced, drive your feet through the ground, and exhale as you push back up and forward to the starting position.

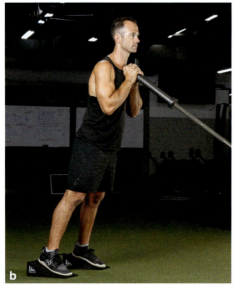

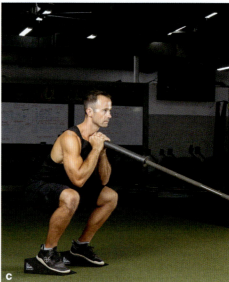

Modifications

Torso lean and foot placement can have a significant impact with this exercise, so, like most squatting movements, you should play with stances and positions to find the position you feel strongest in. Once you find this position, you can modify your torso lean to create more or less horizontal force production (see discussion in chapters 1 and 2 for potential benefits of this). This movement could also be finished on the toes to integrate the calves and triple extension (d).

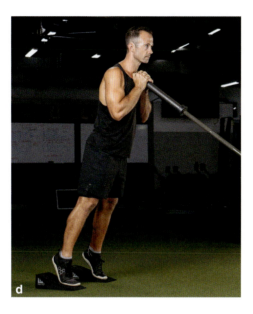

Tips

- Interlace your fingers and keep the wrists tight together against the chest to maintain a solid rack position.
- As weights get heavier, lifting the landmine from the floor to the starting position can become challenging. We recommend using a spotter or elevated starting position when possible.

OFFSET SQUAT

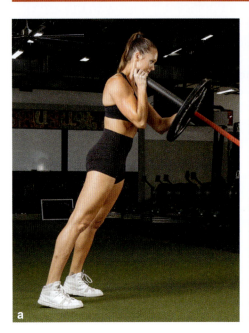
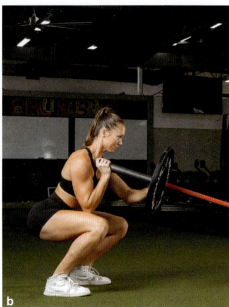

Muscles Targeted

This exercise targets the quads, glutes, and lateral muscles of the core.

Starting Position

Assume a comfortable squatting stance, feet approximately hip width apart and with weight in the balls of the feet so the body is leaned into the landmine. The end of the landmine should be held firmly with the right hand so the forearm is stacked vertically and the elbow is tight to the ribcage. Place the left hand on the weight plate for stability (a).

Coaching Cues

- Allow the weight to shift from the toes into the midfoot as you lower the hips back and down to a parallel (or just below) position (b).
- Brace your core and drive the feet through the ground to return to the starting position.
- Perform the desired number of reps and repeat on the opposite side.

Modifications

Decreasing the depth or elevating the heels to accommodate ankle mobility issues may be an appropriate modification for this exercise. You may also opt out of using the opposite hand for stability, as pictured.

Tips

- Pay attention to the symmetry of your squat and do your best to not allow the offset weight to shift your body to one side.
- We also advise playing with the degree of torso lean to allow you to find what feels like your strongest position with this exercise.

HACK SQUAT

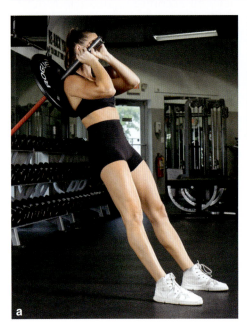 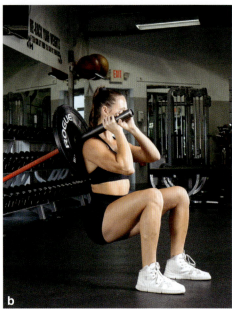

Muscles Targeted

This exercise targets the quads and glutes.

Starting Position

Facing away from the landmine anchor, place the end of the barbell securely on one shoulder with your back up against the weight plate. Toes should be pointing forward with feet in line with the hips. Lean back significantly into the weight plate to allow for proper depth (a).

Coaching Cues

- Use both hands to pull the end of the barbell tight into your body and brace the core before the exercise.
- Bend the knees to slowly lower down into a deep, knee-dominant squat position (b).
- Brace the core and the drive feet through the ground to return to the starting position.
- Perform the desired number of reps and repeat on the opposite side or alternate loaded sides each set.

Modifications

Torso angle will vary from person to person, so play with your body angle to find the position that feels strongest and allows for the greatest depth without compromising form.

Tips

- Make sure to only perform this squat variation with a secure landmine anchor— one that is bolted to the ground or a home base–style attachment placed against the wall so the anchor doesn't slide.
- This exercise can be difficult to set up with heavy loads, so, for safety reasons, it is likely not a great choice for maximal strength training.

OFFSET SURFER SQUAT

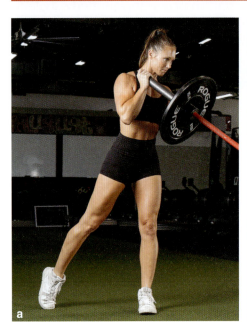
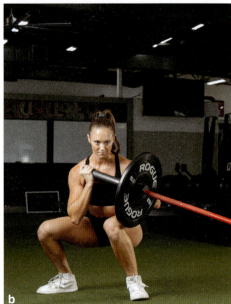

Muscles Targeted

This exercise targets the glutes, quads, hamstrings, and calves.

Starting Position

Grip the landmine in your right hand tight to the shoulder with the left hand supporting farther down the collar. Angle the hips and shoulder approximately 45 degrees away from the landmine anchor. Lean into the barbell with the right heel up off of the ground *(a)*.

Coaching Cues

• Slowly shift your weight and bend down into the right leg so that the heel comes to the floor and your weight shifts back into a squatting motion on the right side *(b)*.

• Drive through the right foot and slightly pivot the foot and hip to return to the starting position.

• Perform the desired number of reps and repeat on the opposite side or alternate loaded sides each set.

Modifications

Stance width can vary based on mobility limitations. This exercise can also be done with more or less rotation in the back foot and hip based on the training goal.

Tips

- Control the descent on this exercise and strive for deeper positions on the back hip to maximize the glutes in this exercise.
- This movement is meant to engage the lateral and rotational motion that the glutes are responsible for, so don't shy away from making it feel athletic.

KICKSTAND SQUAT

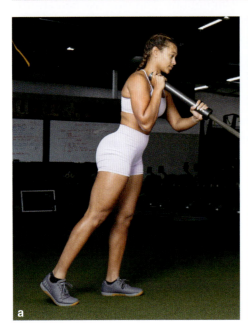
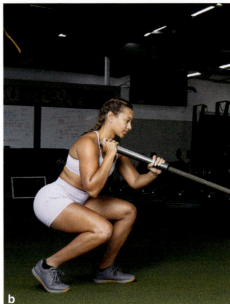

Muscles Targeted

This exercise targets the quads, glutes, and hamstrings.

Starting Position

Grip the landmine in your right hand tight to the shoulder with the left hand supporting farther down the collar. Stance should be hip width with hips facing directly toward the landmine anchor point with a forward lean into the barbell. Right foot is placed just barely behind the left with the heel off of the ground (a).

Coaching Cues

- Sit the left hip back and bend the knee to lower into a deep squat stance while keeping the right heel off of the ground (b).
- Drive up and forward through both feet to return to the starting position.
- Perform the desired number of reps and repeat on the opposite side or alternate loaded sides each set.

Modifications

Depth can be decreased or body angle modified to work around ankle mobility restrictions. This exercise can also be performed using the technique as shown but with both heels off the ground for a more athletic training application *(c)*.

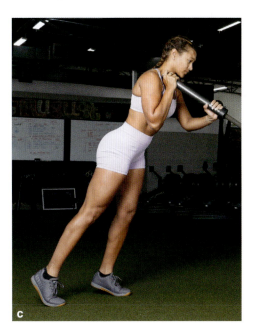

Tips

- As loads increase in the exercise, make sure to pull the barbell in tightly to the torso with the upper body by pulling down onto it and trapping it to the body. This will increase core stability and maintain focus on the upper body.

SISSY SQUAT

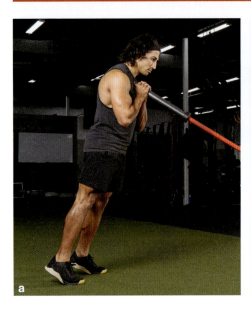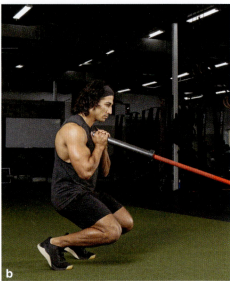

Muscles Targeted

This exercise targets the quadriceps.

Starting Position

Grasp the end of the barbell firmly with both hands while interlocking the fingers. Stand tall with your weight shifted into the balls of the feet and a slight lean into the bar. The bar should be resting along the midline of the collarbone *(a)*.

Coaching Cues

- From a tall position and while maintaining a solid brace, descend by allowing the knees to flex forward while maintaining strict posture between the knees, hips, and shoulders. Lower as far as comfortable or until you feel an appropriate activation of the quads *(b)*.
- Allow the balls of your feet to become the pivot point to send you down. Don't be afraid to push inward toward the landmine to create increased stability within the upper body.
- Push through the balls of the feet to drive back up to the starting position.

Modifications

This exercise demands a lot of the quadriceps, so, initially, less is more with range of motion—listen to your body and don't go for full depth the first time trying this exercise. The goal of this exercise is not to get to the ground but to emphasize movement at the knee and demand on the quads.

Tips

- Unless you have preexisting knee issues, this exercise is considered safe, but be sure to progress range of motion slowly. Chances are most people will not need any additional weight to begin and likely won't touch their knees to the ground.
- Just focus on keeping weight in the balls of the feet and driving a little forward movement of the knees and you will get plenty of quad training stimulus.

SQUAT WITH SIDESTEP

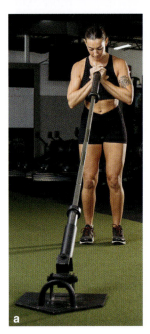 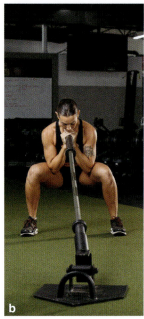 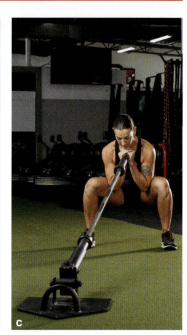

Muscles Targeted

This exercise could be considered full body because of the front-loaded demand on the core, but it primarily targets the quadriceps, upper back, and glutes.

Starting Position

Interlace your fingers to securely grip the far end of the landmine held tightly against the sternum. Place your feet close together directly under the hips and assume a slight lean into the landmine. Weight should be shifted forward slightly into the balls of the feet *(a)*.

Coaching Cues

- Inhale and brace your core with arms held tight to the body.
- Step out to the side with your right foot and simultaneously break at the hips and knees to slowly drop back and down into the bottom squat position, ideally with thighs parallel to the ground *(b)*.
- Keep core braced, drive your feet through the ground, and exhale as you push back up to the starting position.
- Repeat the same step and sequence to the left side *(c)*.

Modifications

Torso lean and foot placement can have a significant impact with this exercise, so, like most squatting movements, you should play with stances and positions to find the position you feel strongest in. There is no one-size-fits-all squatting stance, so hone in on where you feel strongest and can train the greatest range of motion. Once you find this position, you can also modify your torso lean to create more or less horizontal force production (see discussion in chapters 1 and 2 for potential benefits of this).

Tips

- Interlace your fingers and keep wrists tight together against the chest to maintain a solid rack position.
- Load this move slowly to get a feel for the instability of having to step with every repetition.

LUNGE EXERCISES

STATIC LATERAL LUNGE

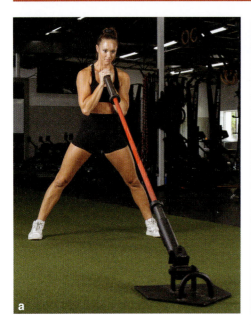

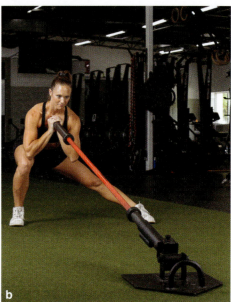

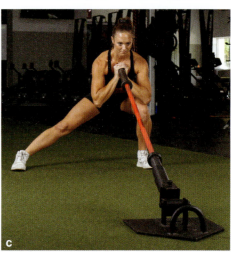

Muscles Targeted

This exercise targets the glutes, hamstrings, quads, and adductors.

Starting Position

Assume a wide stance (at least double hip width) with toes facing forward at the end of the landmine. Interlace your fingers to cradle the end of the barbell and stand tall with the barbell held right in front of the chest (a).

Coaching Cues

- Shift your weight laterally and sit your hips back and to the right while maintaining a straight left leg (b).
- Drive up and back to the left to return to the start position.
- Perform the exercise as described but to the left side (c).

Modifications

Depth and stance on this exercise will be dictated by mobility and limb length. This exercise can also be performed for all repetitions on one side before switching to the opposite leg.

Tips

- As long as the spine is kept relatively straight, don't be afraid to allow for a forward torso lean. The landmine is likely to pull it forward, and this will allow for better hip and glute focus.
- Although not pictured, this exercise could also be held down in front of the body with a similar grip to the forward-facing RDL pictured later in this chapter.

LATERAL LUNGE

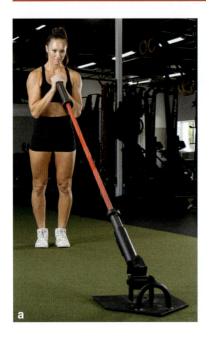 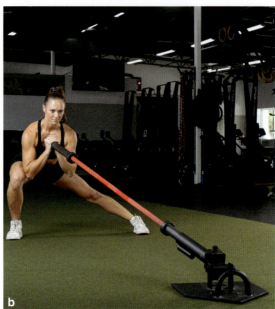

Muscles Targeted

This exercise targets the glutes, quads, hamstrings, and adductors.

Starting Position

Cradle the end of the landmine with both hands held tight to the sternum and stand tall at the end of the bar with both feet together *(a)*.

Coaching Cues

- Step wide to the right and sit your hips back while maintaining a straight left leg *(b)*.
- Drive up and back to the left to return to start position.
- Perform the exercise as described but to the left side.

Modifications

Depth and stance on this exercise will be dictated by mobility and limb length. This exercise can also be performed by stepping onto a slightly elevated surface, such as a box or weight plate, to increase range of motion in the focus leg. However, if performed as described, it should be done one side at a time.

Tips

- Focus on a soft landing for the moving leg to better control the momentum of the landmine.
- Also, progress the width of your lateral step slowly to maintain perfect technique as you drive back up to the starting position.

TOP-LOADED REVERSE LUNGE

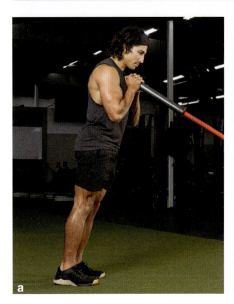 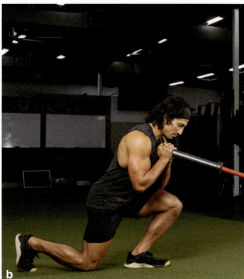

Muscles Targeted

This exercise targets the quads, glutes, and hamstrings.

Starting Position

Interlace the fingers to hold the far end of the landmine securely against the chest. Stand tall with a slight lean into the bar and feet flat on the ground stacked directly under the hips *(a)*.

Coaching Cues

- Keep the landmine and elbows tight to the body to create core tension.
- Slowly step back with the right foot as you allow the left hip and knee to bend and lower to an appropriate bottom position *(b)*.
- Maintain more weight in the left leg and drive through the foot to bring your body back up to the starting position.
- Perform all reps on one side and then repeat on the opposing leg.

Modifications

This exercise serves as the parent position for a handful of progressions (some of which follow); the modifications have a lot to do with range of motion, load placement, and foot placement. The version shown here maintains a stable flat foot on the working leg, but it can also be performed at a greater angle with the front heel elevated off of the ground *(c)*. This move can also be loaded on the opposing shoulder if you're looking to go heavier or to take the upper body out of the equation *(d)*.

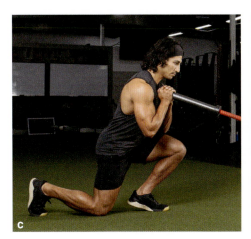 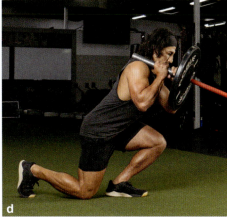

Tips

• You should have a little bit of a forward torso lean that runs parallel to the front shin throughout the movement. If you feel too much tension in the back leg, then shift more weight into the front foot.

• Build strength by performing all reps on one leg before switching. If you wish to challenge your stability and conditioning, alternate legs every repetition for the desired reps.

VARIATION: STEP-THROUGH REVERSE LUNGE

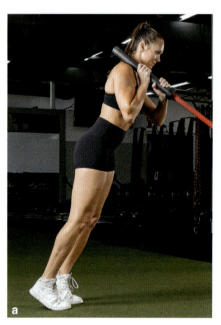
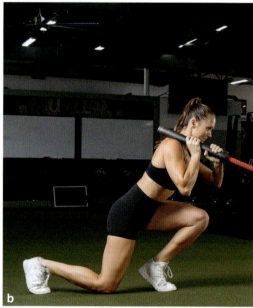

Muscles Targeted

This exercise targets the quads, glutes, hamstrings, and calves.

Starting Position

Rest the far end of the landmine on your right shoulder while holding it closely to the body with the right hand. Place the left hand farther in on the barbell or on the loaded weight plates to stabilize. Walk the feet back to assume a healthy forward lean and come higher up onto the balls of the feet to keep the heels off of the floor *(a)*.

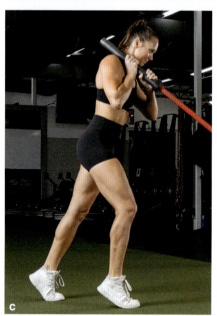

Coaching Cues

- Slowly step back and down with the right foot while allowing the left hip and knee to bend and lower the body to an appropriate bottom position *(b)*.

- While keeping the left heel off of the ground and weight in the left leg, drive through the ball of the foot to bring the body back up and forward toward the landmine.

- The right foot should then step just past the starting position to allow for additional ankle and hip drive from the working leg *(c)*.

Modifications

This exercise is a progression of the top-loaded reverse lunge, so it can be regressed, as needed. Although not pictured, this technique could also be performed in the elevated reverse lunge for even greater range of motion.

Tips

- Torso lean will have a big impact on where you "feel" this one most. Play with a few positions to see where you feel strongest and to target different regions.
- Accentuate the drive up through the ankle at the top of each rep to get a calf burn.
- Perform all reps on the same side for this exercise before changing legs.

VARIATION: ELEVATED REVERSE LUNGE

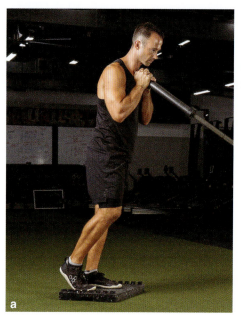 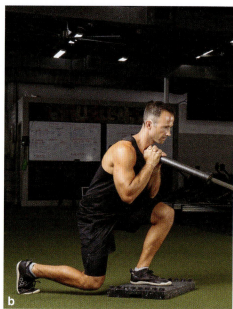

Muscles Targeted

This exercise targets the quads, glutes, and hamstrings.

Starting Position

Interlace the fingers to hold the far end of the landmine securely against the chest. Stand tall on a slightly elevated surface with a slight lean into the bar and feet flat on the ground stacked directly under the hips *(a)*.

Coaching Cues

- Keep the landmine and elbows tight to the body to create core tension.
- Slowly step back with the right foot as you allow the left hip and knee to bend and lower down as low as possible without losing form *(b)*.
- Maintain more weight in the left leg and drive through the foot to bring your body back up to the starting position.
- Perform all reps on one side and then repeat on the opposing leg.

Modifications

This is a progression from the top-loaded reverse lunge, so it can be regressed for a smaller range of motion. The version shown here maintains a stable flat foot on the working leg, but it can also be performed at a greater angle with the front heel elevated off of the ground *(c)*. This move can also be loaded on the opposing shoulder if you're looking to go heavier or to take the upper body out of the equation.

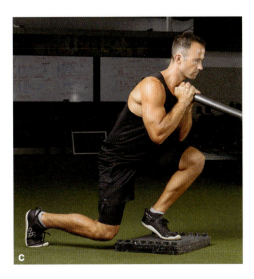

Tips

- You should have a little bit of a forward torso lean that runs parallel to the front shin throughout the movement. If you feel too much tension in the back leg, then shift more weight into the front foot.
- Build strength by performing all reps on one leg before switching. If you wish to challenge your stability and conditioning, alternate legs every repetition for the desired reps.
- For best results, opt for a very short plyometric box or even a 45-pound Olympic plate when choosing an elevated surface.

VARIATION: OVERHEAD REVERSE LUNGE

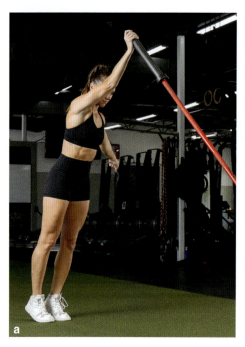
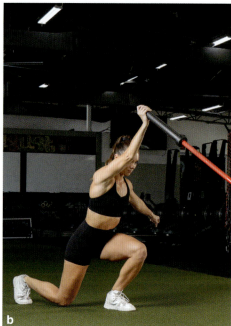

Muscles Targeted

This exercise targets the quads, glutes, and hamstrings, as well as the core with the overhead-loaded position.

Starting Position

Align the right hip with the landmine and maintain a slight lean toward the landmine with the body standing tall. Hold the landmine securely with the right hand and arm locked out fully up and out overhead *(a)*.

Coaching Cues

- Keep the arm holding the landmine tightly locked out and create a fist with the free hand to enhance stability.
- Slowly step back with the right foot as you allow the left hip and knee to bend and lower down as low as possible without losing control of the bar *(b)*.
- Maintain more weight in the left leg and drive through the foot to bring your body back up to the starting position.
- Perform all reps on one side and then repeat on the opposing leg.

Modifications

This is a stability progression from the top-loaded reverse lunge, so make sure to build some movement confidence first, as well as overhead pressing strength, before introducing this exercise. If the instability is too great, then bring the bar back down to the shoulder.

Tips

- Don't try to set any personal records here; use this exercise to improve stability and coordination. This means going for lighter loads and slower tempos.
- Make sure to brace the core and squeeze the nonworking hand to radiate as much tension as needed to control the long lever of the bar overhead.

BOTTOM-LOADED REVERSE LUNGE

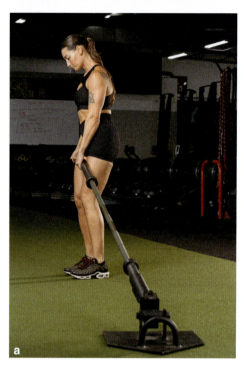
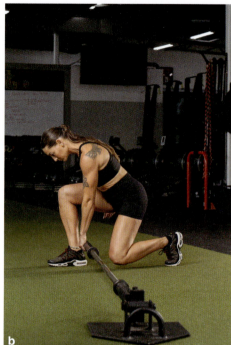

Muscles Targeted

This exercise targets the glutes, hamstrings, and quads.

Starting Position

Stand tall parallel to the landmine anchor with both feet stacked directly underneath the hips. Hold the landmine in your left hand with an overhand grip in front of the left thigh (a).

Coaching Cues

- Keep a tight grip on the landmine and brace the core before beginning the exercise.
- Slowly step back with the left foot while allowing the right hip and knee to bend and lower the body down into a bottom position with a slightly forward torso (b).
- Drive through the entire right foot to bring the body back up to the starting position.
- Perform all reps on one side and then repeat on the opposing leg.

Modifications

Grip can be a limiting factor with this exercise due to the large diameter of the barbell collar, so, if available, use one of the landmine handles mentioned in chapter 2 for heavier loading. This exercise can also be done from an elevated surface, similar to the elevated reverse lunge, for greater range of motion at the hip (c).

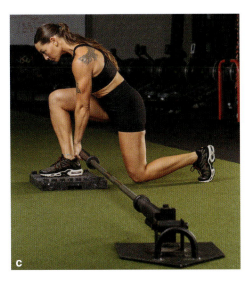

Tips

- Spacing of your body relative to the landmine is key here, so make sure that at the bottom of the lunge your hand and the end of the landmine come just barely inside and above the opposite ankle.
- You should also strive to have a significant forward torso lean as you approach the bottom position to engage the glutes and hamstrings.

ANGLED LANDMINE REVERSE LUNGE

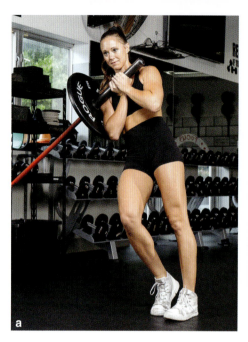
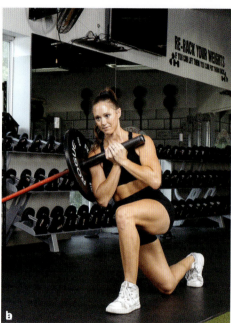

Muscles Targeted

This exercise targets the glutes, hamstrings, and quads.

Starting Position

Stand parallel to the landmine anchor with both feet stacked directly underneath the hips and right shoulder leaning into the loaded weight plates. Hold the landmine in your right hand held securely to the body and hand under the chin. Place the left hand over the top of the right hand to support the weight of the bar (a).

Coaching Cues

• Keep a tight grip on the landmine and brace the core before the exercise.

• While maintaining a significant lean into the landmine, step back with the right foot to allow the left hip and knee to bend and lower down as deep as possible (b).

• Drive through the ball of the foot and outside of the left foot to bring the body back up to the starting position.

• Perform all reps on one side and then repeat on the opposing leg.

Modifications

This exercise can also be performed with what's commonly known as the Zercher position, but we find it to be less comfortable for most exercisers. Once confidence and strength have been built, this exercise, much like the top-loaded reverse lunge, can serve as the foundation for a handful of progressions.

- You can increase range of motion with a slightly elevated surface *(c)*.
- You can create a more athletic application by finishing on the ball of the foot *(d)*.
- You can bring in more lateral motion and the glutes with more of a curtsey stance (see the split squat).

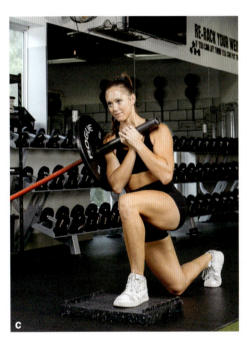
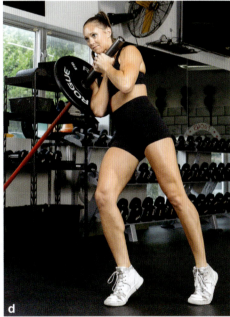

Tips

- Spacing of your body relative to the landmine is key, so try a few different torso angles to find an ideal training stance.
- Also, make sure you are using a landmine anchor that is bolted to the ground or rack or at least wedged into the wall so there is no risk of it sliding as you lean into the anchor point.

SPLIT SQUAT

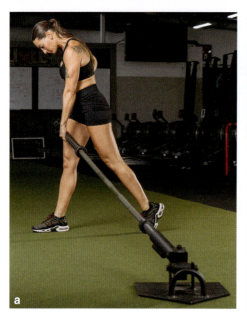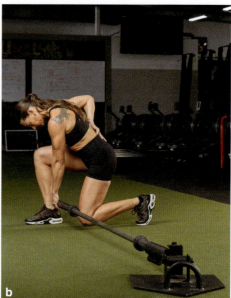

Muscles Targeted

This exercise targets the glutes, quads, and hamstrings.

Starting Position

Stand tall in a split stance parallel to the landmine anchor with the right foot forward. Hold the landmine in your left hand with an overhand grip in front of the left thigh *(a)*.

Coaching Cues

- Keep a tight grip on the landmine and brace the core before the exercise.
- Slowly drop the back knee down and allow the right hip and knee to bend and lower the body down into a bottom position with a slightly forward torso *(b)*.
- Drive through the entire right foot to bring the body back up to the starting position with both legs closed to locked out at the top.
- Perform all reps on one side and then repeat on the opposing leg.

Modifications

Grip can be a limiting factor with this exercise due to the large diameter of the barbell collar; if available, use one of the landmine handles mentioned in chapter 2 for heavier loading. This exercise can also be progressed with the front foot elevated (FFE) and rear foot elevated (RFE) exercises presented in this chapter, both of which increase the range of motion of the exercise.

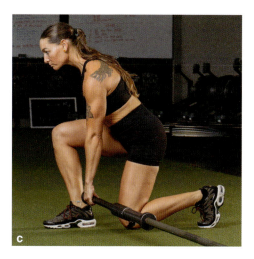

Tips

- Torso angle and the distance between your feet can affect the muscles used.
- A more upright torso will tend to bias more quadriceps (c), while a slight forward lean will target more glute in the front leg.

VARIATION: FRONT FOOT ELEVATED (FFE) SPLIT SQUAT

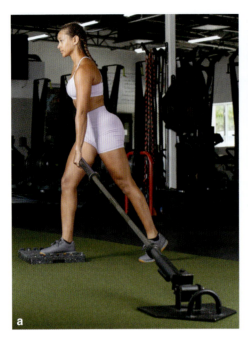
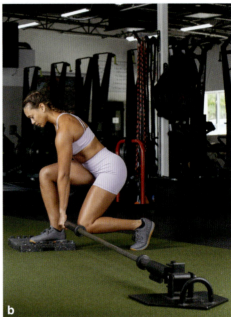

Muscles Targeted

This exercise targets the quads and glutes. If you're new to this variation, it may feel more demanding on the quads compared to the split squat and RFE split squat.

Starting Position

Stand tall in a split stance parallel to the landmine anchor with the right foot forward on a slightly elevated surface. Hold the landmine in your left hand with an overhand grip in front of the left thigh (a).

Coaching Cues

- Keep a tight grip on the landmine and brace the core before the exercise.
- Slowly shift forward and allow both knees to bend to lower the body into a deep bottom position with a slight forward lean (b).
- Drive through the entire right foot and straighten both legs to return to a relatively locked-out position at the top.
- Perform all reps on one side and then repeat on the opposing leg.

Modifications

This exercise is a range-of-motion progression from the split squat, so regress to lessen the range of motion, as needed. It may also be performed with an alternate handle for those limited by grip *(c)*.

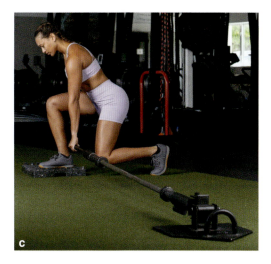

Tips

- Torso angle and the distance between your feet can also affect the muscles used.
- It's preferable to have a slight forward lean to bias more of the front leg during the exercise and to lessen pressure on the hip flexors and quads on the rear leg.

REAR FOOT ELEVATED (RFE) SPLIT SQUAT

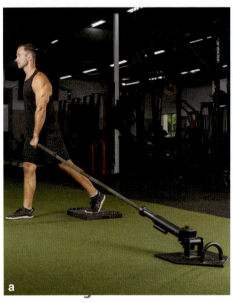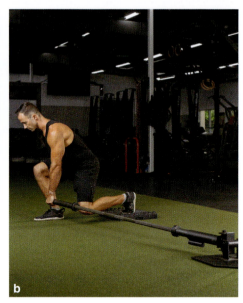

This exercise targets the glutes, quads, and hamstrings.

Starting Position

Stand tall in a split stance parallel to the landmine anchor with the right foot forward and left foot placed back on a slightly elevated surface. Hold the landmine in your left hand with an overhand grip more in line with the right leg and weight shifted slightly forward (a).

Coaching Cues

- Keep a tight grip on the landmine and brace the core before the exercise.
- Slowly drop the back knee down, allowing both knees to bend and lowering into a deep bottom position with a slight forward lean (b).
- Drive through the entire right foot and straighten both legs to return to a relatively locked-out position at the top.
- Perform all reps on one side and then repeat on the opposing leg.

Modifications

This exercise is a great regression from the full Bulgarian split squat *(c)*, so start small with the height of the step and progress it slowly. Higher surfaces will increase range of motion in the front leg and can slightly change the setup position.

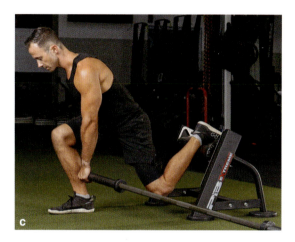

Tips

• Maintain a slight forward lean (as pictured) to emphasize range of motion at the front hip on this exercise.

• While performing the exercise, you want to feel like you have more weight in the front working leg throughout.

BULGARIAN SPLIT SQUAT

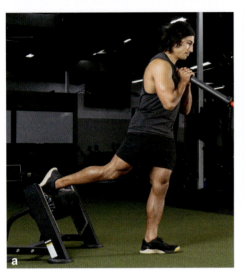 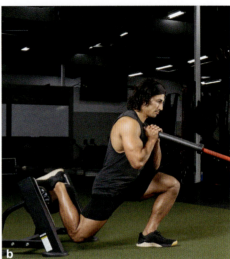

Muscles Targeted

This exercise targets the glutes, quads, and hamstrings.

Starting Position

Stand tall facing the landmine anchor with the end of the barbell cradled in the hands tight to the chest. Take a step back with the right foot to place the shoelaces lightly on top of a split squat stand or bench. Keep your weight centered on the front foot and maintain a slight forward lean of the torso *(a)*.

Coaching Cues

- Keep a tight grip on the landmine and brace the core before the exercise.
- Slowly drop the back knee down to allow for the body to shift backward and down into a strong bottom position *(b)*.
- Drive through the entire left foot to bring the body back up and forward into the starting position.
- Perform all reps on one side and then repeat on the opposing leg.

Modifications

This exercise can also be performed with more of an offset load and the end of the landmine resting on the shoulder *(c)*.

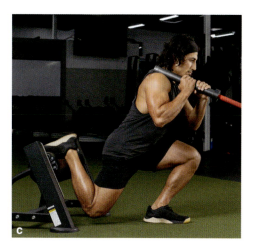

Tips

• Make sure not to elevate the back foot on a surface that is higher than the bottom of the knee when standing. Doing so can create too much tension on the rear nonworking leg.

• Also, be conscious of feeling more weight in the front foot throughout and only go as deep as you can maintain technique, as pictured.

HINGE EXERCISES

FORWARD-FACING RDL

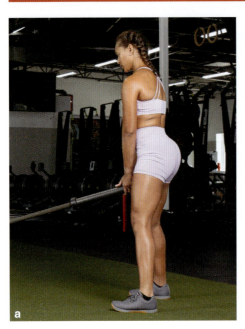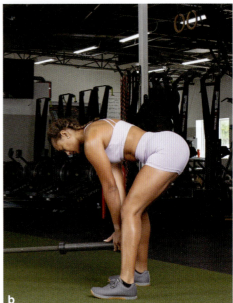

Muscles Targeted

This exercise targets the glutes, hamstrings, and low back.

Starting Position

Stand tall facing the landmine anchor with the end of the barbell cradled in the hands just in front of the hips. Feet should be right around hip width with toes relatively forward (a).

Coaching Cues

- Take a big breath and brace the core as you initiate the downward phase of the exercise.
- Maintaining a slight bend in the knees, push the hips back to allow the body to slowly come down so the wrists just pass the knees (b).
- Maintain core tension and push your feet back through the ground to return to a good starting position.

Modifications

The general setup is described above, but playing with the distance between the feet and the landmine may be appropriate for some exercisers. The exercise can also be safely performed from wider stances (see adductor RDL) for those looking to involve more inner thigh activation.

Tips

- Don't compromise low back position for depth in this exercise. Only go as low as you can maintain the same spinal alignment throughout the exercise.
- Also, don't fall into the technique mistake of trying to lift your toes off the ground to get more hamstrings. Maintaining toe contact on the ground throughout the exercise will allow for better strength and glute recruitment throughout the movement.

REAR-FACING RDL

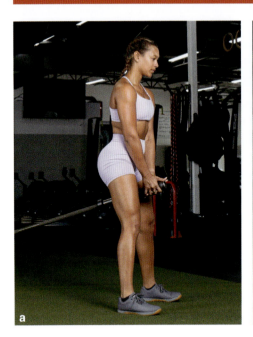
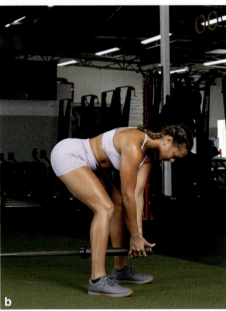

Muscles Targeted

This exercise targets the glutes, hamstrings, and low back.

Starting Position

Stand tall facing away from the landmine anchor and gripping a smaller weight plate (or handle attachment) in front of the hips with both hands. Your body should be upright but your weight should feel like it's shifted slightly back into the landmine (a).

Coaching Cues

- Take a big breath and pull the weight plate into the body to engage the lats before starting the movement.
- Maintaining a slight bend in the knees, push the hips back to allow your hips to hinge and slowly lower until your hands are in line with the middle of the shin (b).
- Maintain core tension and push your feet back through the ground to return to a good starting position.

Modifications

This is a great variation to go to if the forward-facing RDL gives you too much discomfort in the low back; the additional lat engagement and body position tend to fix this for most people. Play with foot placement closer to or farther away from the anchor to accommodate as well.

Tips

• We recommend using weight plates, or an additional handle attachment for better hand position, but a towel wrapped around the bar with a secure landmine anchor point can also work.

• Although weight placement is different in this setup than with the forward-facing variation, we recommend keeping the toes down and feet firmly placed on the ground.

ADDUCTOR RDL

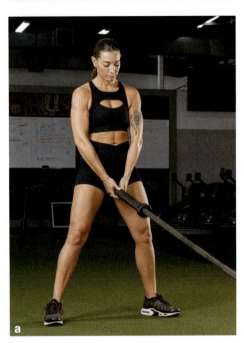
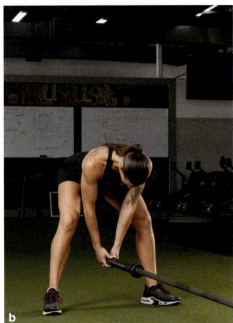

Muscles Targeted

This exercise targets the hamstring, adductors, and glutes.

Starting Position

Stand tall facing the landmine anchor with the end of the barbell cradled in the hands just in front of the hips. Feet should be at least double hip width and toes turned slightly out *(a)*.

Coaching Cues

- Take a big breath and brace the core as you initiate the downward phase of the exercise.
- Maintaining a slight bend in the knees, push the hips back to allow the body to slowly come down so the wrists just pass the knees *(b)*.
- Maintain core tension and push your feet back through the ground to return to a good starting position.

Modifications

If greater depth is desired, then use smaller weight plates to increase the distance to the ground you can travel or elevate the feet off the ground *(c)*.

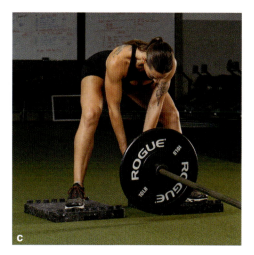

Tips

- Don't compromise low back position for depth in this exercise. Only go as low as you can maintain the same spinal alignment throughout the exercise.
- Feet should remain flat on the ground throughout the exercise. It's normal to feel slightly more weight on the outside of the foot based on the wide stance.

STAGGERED RDL

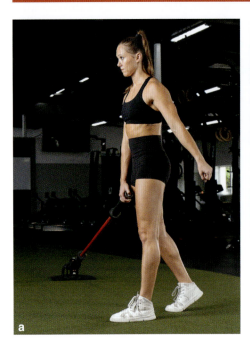
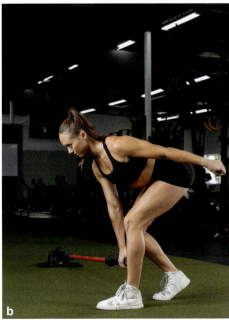

Muscles Targeted

This exercise targets the glutes, hamstrings, and lower back muscles.

Starting Position

Stand parallel to the landmine anchor with the end of the barbell held in the right hand against the right thigh. Align the ball of the right foot with the heel of the left to assume a staggered stance. Weight should be shifted into the left foot with the right heel off of the ground (a).

Coaching Cues

- Take a big breath and brace the core as you initiate the downward phase of the exercise.
- Maintaining a slight bend in the left knee, push the hips back to bring the torso down until the right hand is in line with the middle of the shin (b).
- Maintain core tension and push back through the left foot to bring the body back to the starting position.
- Perform all reps on one side and then repeat on the opposing leg.

Modifications

Foot placement and depth in the exercise may vary based on build and flexibility. This exercise can also be performed with a purposeful lateral lean into the barbell to bring in more abductors *(c)*.

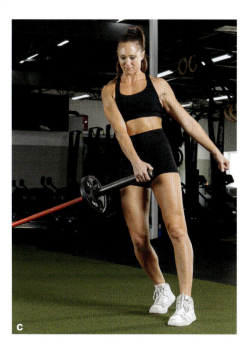

Tips

- Try not to let the barbell rotate you during the exercise.
- As for spacing, the barbell should also come right down on top of and inside the shoelaces to maintain appropriate loading of the hamstrings and glutes.

STEPPING RDL

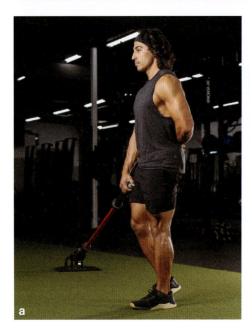 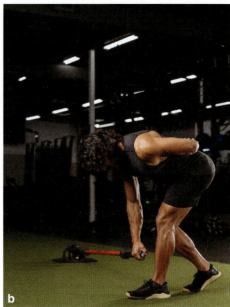

Muscles Targeted

This exercise targets the glutes, hamstrings, and lower back muscles.

Starting Position

Stand angled in just slightly off of parallel to the landmine anchor with the end of the barbell held in the right hand against the right thigh. Weight should be shifted into the left foot with the right foot lightly on the ground *(a)*.

Coaching Cues

- Take a big breath and brace the core as you initiate the downward phase of the exercise.
- Maintain a slight lean of the body into the landmine and step back to bring the right foot just behind the left and shift the hips back to bring the torso down until the right hand is in line with the middle of the shin *(b)*.
- Maintain core tension and push back through the ball of the foot to bring the body back to the starting position.
- Perform all reps on one side and then repeat on the opposing leg.

Modifications

This exercise may feel more natural with both hands holding the end of the landmine due to the lateral lean of the barbell *(c)*.

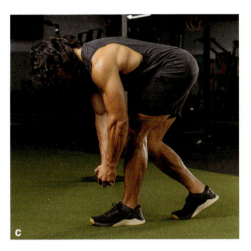

Tips

- Make the step with the back foot feel very light to maintain tension on the working lead leg.
- It may be hard to see, but ever so slightly turn the toe of the working leg inward toward the landmine to maximize hip extension and abduction—the two major roles of your glutes!

SINGLE-LEG RDL

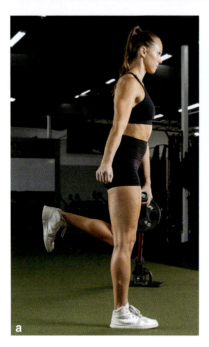
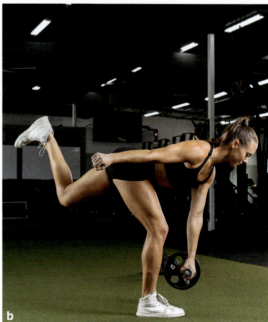

Muscles Targeted

This exercise targets the glutes, hamstrings, and lower back muscles.

Starting Position

Stand parallel to the landmine anchor with the end of the barbell held in the left hand against the left thigh. Weight should be shifted into the right foot with the left knee bent to 90 degrees and off of the floor *(a)*.

Coaching Cues

- Take a big breath and brace the core as you initiate the downward phase of the exercise.
- Maintain a soft bend in the right knee and push the hips back to bring the torso down until the left hand is in line with the middle of the shin *(b)*.
- Maintain core tension and drive through the entire right foot to bring the body back up to the starting position.
- Perform all reps on one side and then repeat on the opposing leg.

Modifications

The landmine aids in balance with this exercise, but if the instability is too much for the working leg, then regress to a staggered RDL position.

Tips

- To avoid the common error of rounding the back, think about driving the foot of the bent leg back and up to the ceiling. This will emphasize movement at the hip rather than reaching down and forward with the landmine.
- Also, make sure to keep the landmine tight to the body.

KNEELING HIP EXTENSION

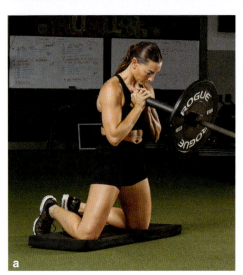
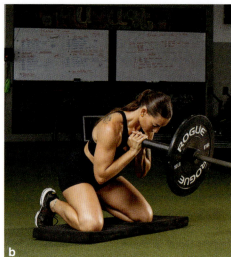

Muscles Targeted

This exercise targets the glutes, lower back, and hamstrings.

Starting Position

Interlace your fingers to securely grip the far end of the landmine held tightly against the sternum. Assume a tall kneeling position with knees slightly wider than the hips and toes dug into the ground. Weight should be shifted forward slightly into the bar (a).

Coaching Cues

- Take a big breath and brace the core as you initiate the downward phase of the exercise.
- Push the hips back toward the heels and allow for the torso to come down slightly toward the ground (b).
- Maintain core tension and drive through the toes to engage the hamstrings and glutes and bring the body back to the starting position.

Modifications

This is the starting point for the kneeling thruster; it can be turned into a full body exercise by adding the explosive press to the hip extension shown here. Although a slightly more involved setup, this exercise can also be intensified with a band *(c)* like the NT Loop for greater glute recruitment.

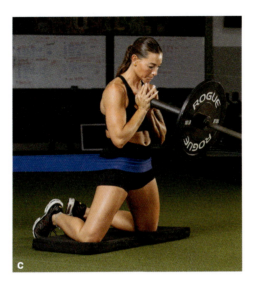

Tips

- This exercise can be loaded relatively heavy and may be easier to set up with one of the elevated starting positions discussed in chapter 2.
- We also recommend making sure you have plenty of padding under the knees.

LANDMINE SUMO DEADLIFT

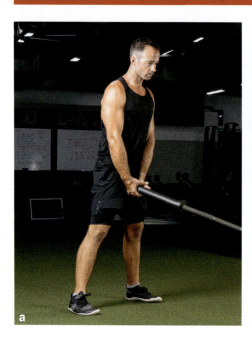
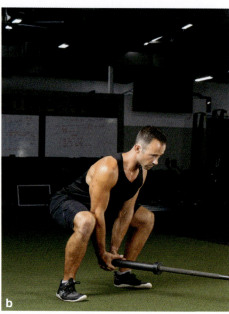

Muscles Targeted

This exercise targets the hamstrings, adductors, and glutes.

Starting Position

Stand tall facing the landmine anchor with the end of the barbell cradled in the hands just in front of the hips. Feet should be at least double hip width and toes turned slightly out *(a)*.

Coaching Cues

- Take a big breath and brace the core as you initiate the downward phase of the exercise.
- Simultaneously break at the hips and knees to sit back into a deep squatlike position *(b)*.
- Maintain core tension and push your feet back through the ground to return to the starting position.

Modifications

The distance between the feet and foot position can be modified to find the stance that feels strongest. Range of motion can also be increased by elevating both feet slightly up off of the ground *(c)*.

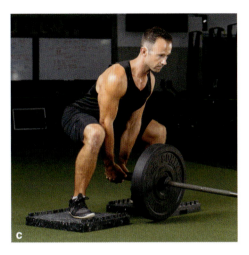

Tips

- This tends to be a very strong lower body stance for most people, so don't be surprised if grip becomes a limiting factor.
- As for position, this should feel like a hybrid between a squat and a deadlift. You want to sit down into it like a squat but maintain a significant hinge at the hips, as pictured.

LOWER BODY ACCESSORY EXERCISES

STANDING CALF RAISE

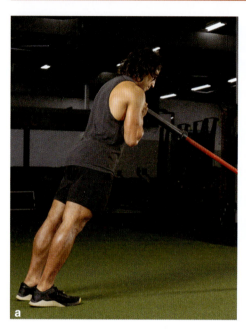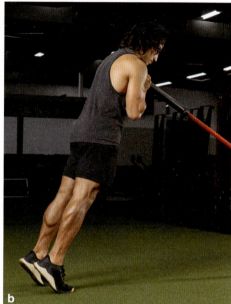

Muscles Targeted

This exercise targets the two main calf muscles: the gastrocnemius and the soleus.

Starting Position

Stand tall facing the landmine anchor with the end of the barbell cradled in the palms held tight against the chest. Assume a hip-width stance and a significant lean into the barbell with feet flat on the ground (a).

Coaching Cues

- Brace the core to maintain tension throughout the exercise.
- From a stretched calf position, drive through the ball of the foot to elevate the body up and forward as much as possible (b).
- Slowly pull the body back down into a fully stretched position for the calves.

Modifications

Body angle can be increased or decreased based on calf flexibility and strength to ensure an adequate full range of motion. Foot position can also be played with (e.g., toes forward, in, or out) to emphasize certain portions of the calf. Lastly, the exercise could be performed from a slightly elevated surface to allow for greater range of motion (c).

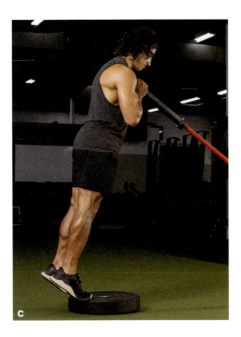

Tips

• Load this one up before feeling the need to elevate, as the unique ability of the landmine to include a forward trajectory will also work the calves in a slightly different way than a traditional standing calf raise.

STAGGERED CALF RAISE

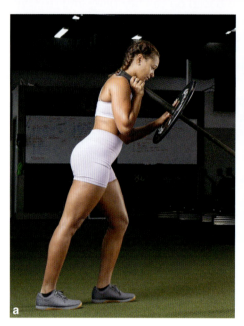 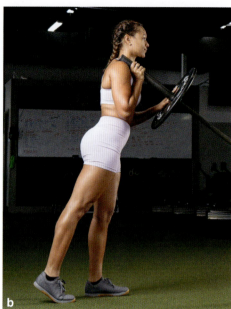

Muscles Targeted

This exercise will smoke your calves.

Starting Position

Stand tall facing the landmine anchor with the end of the barbell resting on the right shoulder. The right leg should be staggered back so the leg is straight and the calf fully stretched. The left foot is placed slightly in front just to maintain balance *(a)*.

Coaching Cues

- Keep 90 percent or more of your weight in the working leg throughout the exercise.
- From a stretched calf position, drive the ball of the foot into the ground, bringing your body up and forward as much as possible *(b)*.
- Slowly pull the body back down into a fully stretched calf position.
- Complete all reps on one side before switching sides.

Modifications

Body angle can be increased or decreased based on calf flexibility and strength to ensure a full range of motion.

Tips

- Exaggerate the forward lean of your body as much as your ankle flexibility will allow to work the full length of the muscle *(c)*.

- Introduce with slow eccentric tempos to gain both strength and flexibility.

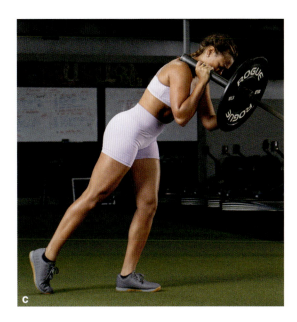

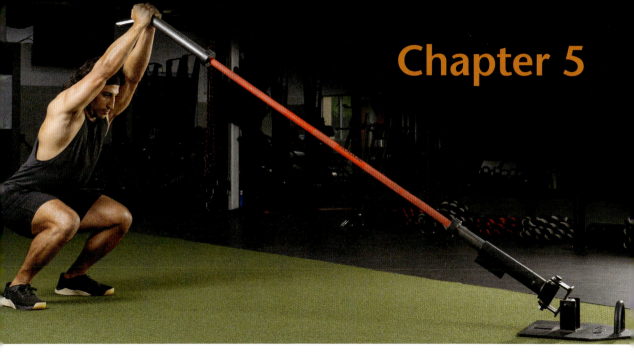

Chapter 5

FULL BODY EXERCISES

This chapter includes landmine exercises geared toward training and challenging the entire body. Many of these movements are combinations of exercises listed in previous chapters or more explosive full body versions. Many of the techniques required for some of the movements are more nuanced, and you will want to ensure that you are building strength and confidence in your ability to perform the movements before combining them into some of the exercises that follow. The exercises in this chapter are listed in order of increasing complexity, so you will have an idea of the skill level each requires. As with all of the exercises in this book, focus on form with lighter loads and slower speeds first to master each move before progressing intensity.

LANDMINE THRUSTER

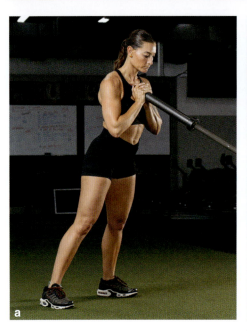

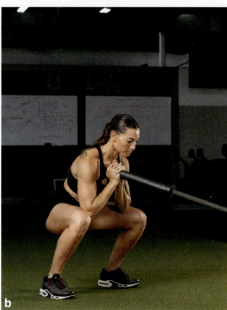

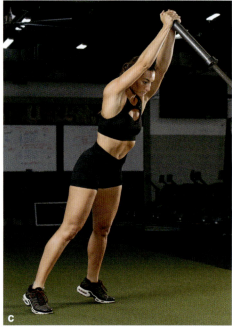

Muscles Targeted

This is a full body exercise, but it does place a lot of load on the glutes, quads, shoulders, and core.

Starting Position

Interlace your fingers to securely grip the far end of the landmine held tightly against the sternum. Place your feet slightly wider than hip width and assume a slight lean into the landmine. Weight should be shifted forward slightly into the balls of the feet *(a)*.

Coaching Cues

- Inhale and brace your core with arms held tight to the body.
- Simultaneously break at the hips and knees to slowly drop back and down into the bottom position, ideally with thighs parallel to the ground *(b)*.
- Keep the core braced, drive your feet through the ground, and exhale as you simultaneously drive the barbell up and forward into an overhead locked-out position *(c)*.
- Control the barbell back down to a starting position and repeat for the desired number of repetitions.

Modifications

Torso lean and foot placement can have a significant effect on this exercise, so, like most squatting movements, you should play with stances and positions to find the position you feel strongest in. Once you find this position, you can also modify your torso lean to create more or less horizontal force production (see discussions in chapters 1 and 2 for potential benefits).

Tips

- Interlace your fingers and keep wrists tight together against the chest to maintain a solid rack position.
- This exercise can be executed with heavier loads and normal tempos for building full body strength or with moderate to lighter loads with explosive concentric (upward) movements to improve power production.
- Make sure you have already developed proficiency with the landmine squat and standing press before combining them with the thruster.

SQUAT JUMP

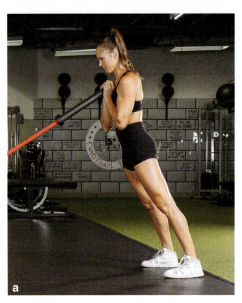

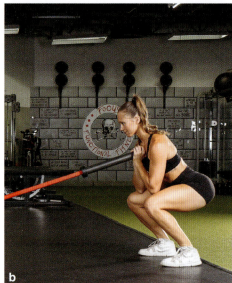

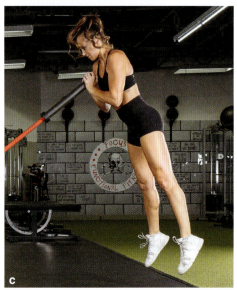

Muscles Targeted

The primary muscles targeted are the glutes and quads, but this exercise was placed in the full body chapter because of the additional load placed on the entire body, including the core and shoulder complex.

Starting Position

Interlace your fingers to securely grip the far end of the landmine held tightly against the sternum. Place your feet slightly wider than hip width and assume a slight lean into the landmine. Weight should be shifted forward slightly into the balls of the feet *(a)*.

Coaching Cues

- Inhale and brace your core with arms held tight to the body.
- Simultaneously break at the hips and knees to drop back and down into the bottom position, ideally with thighs parallel to the ground or slightly above *(b)*.
- Keep the core braced, drive your feet through the ground, and explode up so that the feet slightly leave the ground *(c)*.
- Softly land and return to the start position and repeat for the desired number of reps.

Modifications

This exercise can also be performed with the same explosive upward intent and not leaving the ground. This can be a great way to gain some of the power benefits of the exercise without the additional impact of jumping.

Tips

- Only after developing strength and proficiency with the landmine squat should the squat jump be integrated into the program to ensure safety and effectiveness.

- Maintain a solid brace and position of the landmine against the sternum so you don't lose out on any power production.

- Start with less than 40 percent of your comfortable landmine goblet squat weight and keep repetitions low to moderate to focus on quality execution.

SQUAT HOLD PRESS

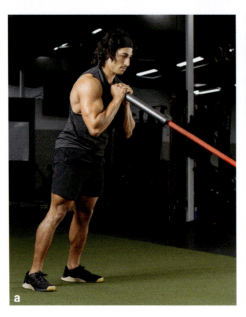

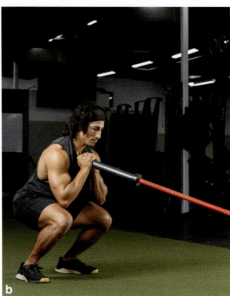

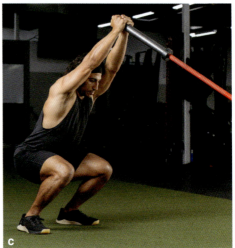

Muscles Targeted

This exercise targets the entire body but is likely most taxing on the shoulders and upper back.

Starting Position

Interlace your fingers to securely grip the far end of the landmine held tightly against the sternum. Place your feet slightly wider than hip width and assume a slight lean into the landmine. Weight should be shifted forward slightly into the balls of the feet (a).

Coaching Cues

- Inhale and brace your core with arms held tight to the body.
- Simultaneously break at the hips and knees to slowly drop back and down into the bottom position, ideally with thighs parallel to the ground (b).
- Keep the core braced and maintain (isometric) the lower body position while driving the landmine up and out overhead (c).

Modifications

Based on ankle and hip flexibility limitations, you may also slightly elevate the heels to maintain a better squat position during the exercise *(d)*.

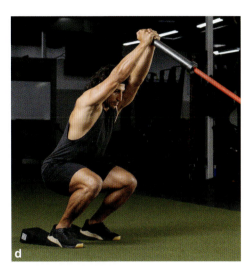

Tips

- This exercise is best suited for building integrity and strength in the upper back in the bottom squat position.
- Think of it as an accessory exercise and prioritize quality movement with lighter loads and slower tempos to get the most out of it.

KNEELING PUSH PRESS

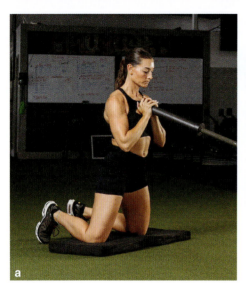
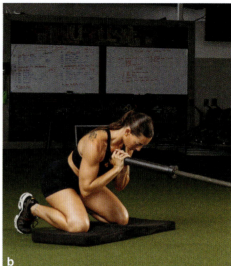
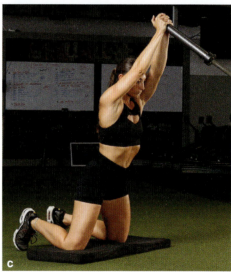

Muscles Targeted

This exercise targets the hip extensors (glutes and low back), as well as the shoulders, triceps, and chest.

Starting Position

Interlace your fingers to securely grip the far end of the landmine held tightly against the sternum. Assume a tall kneeling position with knees on the ground slightly wider than hip width and toes dug into the ground (a).

Coaching Cues

- Inhale and brace your core with arms held tight to the body.

- Break at the hips and hinge so the butt comes back towards the heels (b).

- Keep the core braced, drive your hips forward, and finish by explosively driving the bar overhead into a locked-out position (c).

- Slowly lower the bar back to the starting position and repeat for the desired number of repetitions.

Modifications

This exercise can also be performed with accommodating band resistance (chapter 2) and with an elevated starting position to more easily set up for the starting position *(d)*.

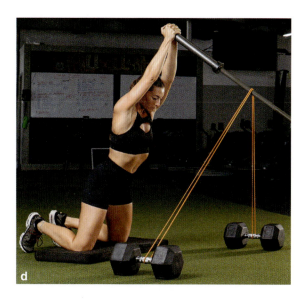

Tips

- Prerequisites to getting the most out of this exercise would be building strength in the lower body hinging and upper body pressing exercises included in earlier chapters.
- When introducing this as a new exercise, focus on a slow descent to maintain core tension and glute engagement to minimize low back strain.

LANDMINE HANG CLEAN

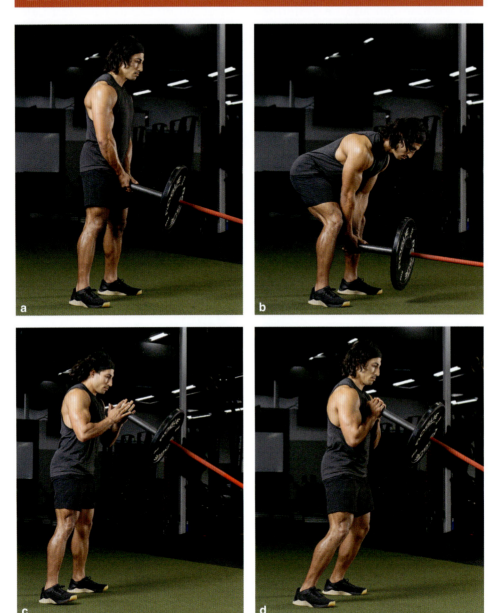

Muscles Targeted

This exercise targets the glutes, hamstrings, and other posterior chain muscles involved in jumping.

Starting Position

Interlace your fingers to cradle the landmine in front of the hips. Assume a stance just wider than hip width with the toes pointed forward *(a)*.

Coaching Cues

- Inhale and brace your core before executing.
- Maintain a soft bend in the knees as you hinge the hips back until the hands come just below the knees *(b)*.
- Keeping the core braced, explode upward so that the bar travels up and momentarily leaves the hands *(c)* as you quickly slide your hands underneath the bar to cradle it with the palms together at chest level *(d)*.
- Control the bar back to the starting position.

Tips

- Execution of this one takes time and starts to integrate a higher level of skill in catching the landmine in the right position. The key is to start light to build the skills and to use bumper plates when available so that any missed catches don't damage the training floor.
- We also recommend this exercise be performed with a secure landmine attachment that will not shift around during the exercise.

SINGLE-ARM CLEAN

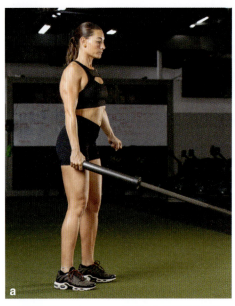
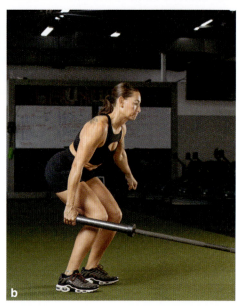
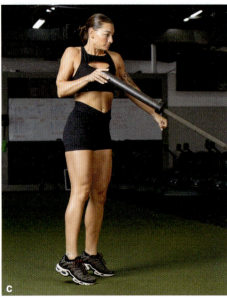
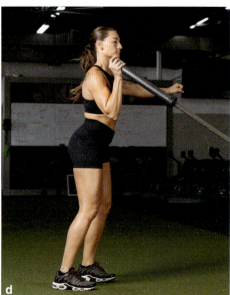

Muscles Targeted

This exercise targets the glutes, hamstrings, and obliques due to the offset loading.

Starting Position

Stand tall with a hip-width stance facing the landmine anchor and holding the far end of the landmine with your right hand next to the thigh (a).

Coaching Cues

- Inhale and brace your core before executing.
- Maintain a soft bend in the knees as you hinge the hips back until the right hand reaches a height just above the knee *(b)*.
- Keep the core braced and explode upward *(c)* so that the bar travels up to chest height while you simultaneously slide your hand under to a shoulder-racked position and safely catch the bar *(d)*.
- Control the bar back to the starting position.

Modifications

This exercise could also be combined to include a press after the coaching cues to form a single-arm clean and press *(e)*. Combine these cues with those from the single-arm press on page 42 in chapter 3.

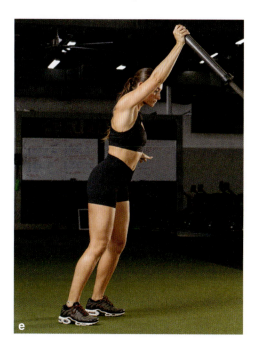

Tips

- Focus on trying to feel explosive and "snappy" in this exercise rather than going for big weights.
- You can also create tension in the opposite hand by making a fist (see photos) to maximize torso and core tension in this exercise.

SINGLE-LEG RDL-TO-ROW

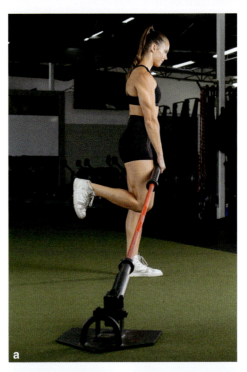

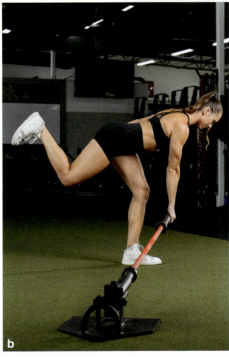

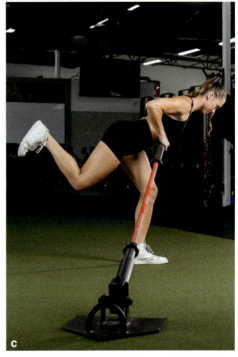

Muscles Targeted

This exercise targets the glutes, lats, and muscles of the low back.

Starting Position

Stand parallel to the landmine anchor with the end of the barbell held in the right hand against the right thigh. Weight should be shifted into the left foot with the right knee bent and the foot off of the floor *(a)*.

Coaching Cues

- Take a big breath and brace the core as you initiate the downward phase of the exercise.
- Maintain a soft bend in the left knee and push the hips back to bring the torso down until the right hand is in line with the middle of the shin and the right leg is in line with the torso *(b)*.
- Maintain core tension and then pull the hand and end of the landmine up and back near the bottom ribs *(c)*.
- Slowly control the arm back down to the bottom position and repeat for the desired number of repetitions before executing on the opposite side.

Modifications

This exercise could be performed isometrically at the hips by performing all of the desired rowing reps while holding the position shown in figure *b*. This is a great way to work on building isometric strength and integrity in the hips. It could also be done in sequence where a full RDL is performed in between each rep to make it feel more like a full body combination-style movement.

Tips

- Lead the exercise by thinking about lifting the back leg back and up to drive the movement at the hip. This is a great way to avoid the "rounding" at the back that often happens with hinging exercises.

REVERSE LUNGE THRUSTER

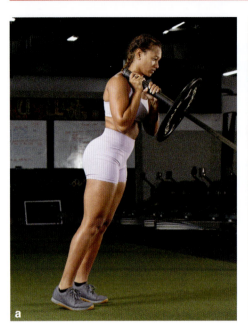

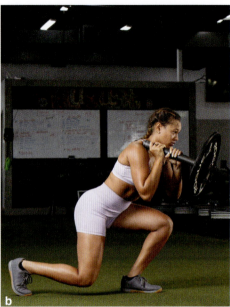

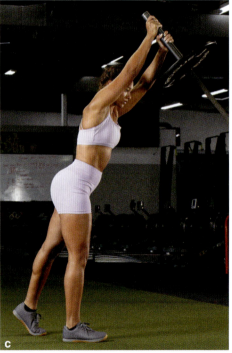

Muscles Targeted

This exercise targets the entire body but is most demanding on the quads, glutes, and shoulders.

Starting Position

Rest the far end of the landmine in your right hand held tight to the shoulder. Place the left hand further in on the barbell to stabilize. Walk the feet back to assume a healthy forward lean and come up onto the balls of the feet *(a)*.

Coaching Cues

- Slowly step back and down with the right foot while allowing the left hip and knee to bend and lower the body to an appropriate bottom position *(b)*.

- While keeping the weight in the left leg, drive through the ball of the foot to bring the body back up while simultaneously driving the landmine overhead with both hands into a locked-out position *(c)*.

- The right foot should then step just past the starting position to allow for additional ankle and hip drive from the working leg.

Modifications

Lunge depth and torso angle can be modified with this exercise based on your goal. If you're looking for more hip power often associated with exercises like jumping (e.g., broad jump), then you may purposefully not step back into full lunge depth but make it slightly more hip dominant. This may also slightly affect your torso angle, which will allow you to create more forward force into the bar.

Tips

- Make sure to master the top-loaded reverse lunge and the standing landmine press exercises separately before combining them into this exercise.

ROTATIONAL SQUAT-TO-PRESS

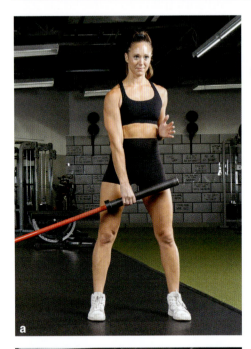

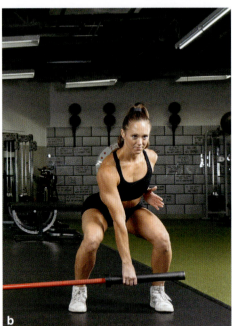

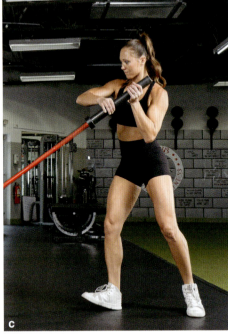

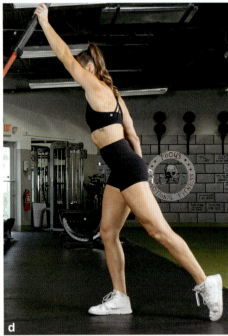

Muscles Targeted

This exercise targets the entire body but is most demanding on the glutes and core.

Starting Position

Standing parallel to the landmine, hold the far end of the landmine with the right hand in front of the hips. Place feet a little wider than hip width than you would normally squat in *(a)*.

Coaching Cues

- Bend the knees and break at the hips to sit down into a squat position with the landmine end centered in between the legs and around shin height *(b)*.
- Explode up and to the right with the landmine by driving off of the left foot and rotating the entire body explosively *(c)* so that you finish the move by driving the landmine up into a locked-out position with the left hand *(d)*.
- The feet should also rotate with the hips to finish the move in a solid split-stance position.

Modifications

You can also perform more of a "hand-off" from one hand to the next instead of letting go to transition, as pictured *(e)*. This is an easier way to get comfortable with the rotational motion and also may allow for more strength versus power programming.

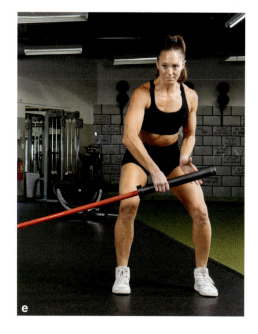

Tips

- When done with much lighter weights, this can be a great functional warm-up exercise because it teaches the body to transfer forces from the lower to the upper body.
- If using it for prep work or strength work, then emphasize slower lowering speeds before transitioning into full-speed explosive versions.

ROTATIONAL RDL-TO-PRESS

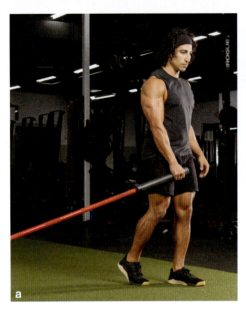
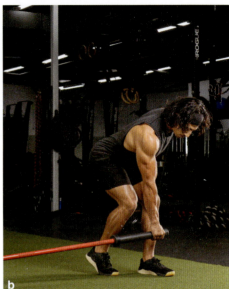

Muscles Targeted

This exercise targets the entire body but is most demanding on the glutes and core.

Starting Position

Standing parallel to the landmine, hold the far end of the landmine with the right hand just inside of the left leg. Place the right foot slightly back to assume a slightly staggered position (a).

Coaching Cues

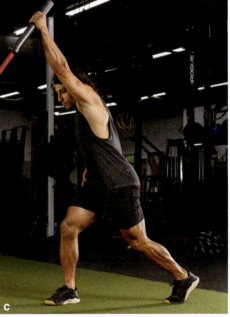

- Maintain a soft bend in the left knee and break at the hips to hinge back until the landmine travels in line with or slightly below the knee (b).

- Explode up and to the right with the landmine by driving off of the left foot and rotating the entire body explosively so that you finish the move by driving the landmine up into a locked-out position with the left hand (c).

- The feet should also rotate with the hips to finish the move in a solid split-stance position.

Modifications

You can also perform more of a "hand-off" from one hand to the next instead of letting go to transition, as shown *(d)*. This is an easier way to get comfortable with the rotational motion and also may allow for more strength versus power programming.

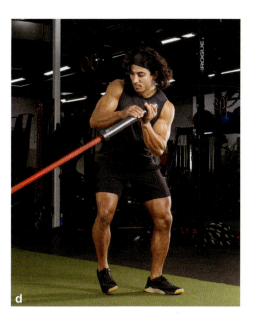

Tips

- When done with much lighter weights, this can be a great functional warm-up exercise because it teaches the body to transfer forces from the lower to the upper body.
- If using it for prep work or strength work, then emphasize slower lowering speeds before transitioning into full-speed explosive versions.

STEP-THROUGH PRESS

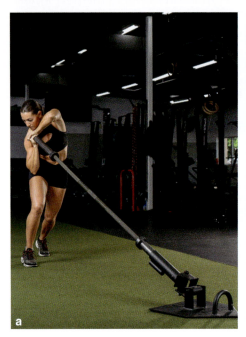 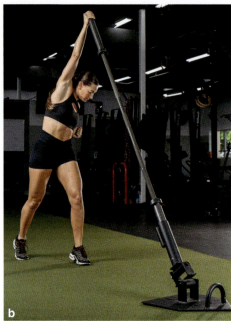

Muscles Targeted

This exercise targets the entire body but is mostly driven by the glutes, core, and shoulders.

Starting Position

Hold the landmine securely at the far end with the right hand near the shoulder and elbow tucked tight to the ribs. The left hand is on top of the right and the left elbow drives up to place the left lats under a slight stretch. Lean into the barbell and assume a staggered stance with the right leg forward and both heels off of the ground *(a)*.

Coaching Cues

- Maintain core tension and a tight coil before initiating the movement.
- Explode forward off of the right foot and simultaneously throw the left elbow behind you to use rotational core power to finish with the right arm locked out overhead *(b)*.
- The left foot should also step forward to finish in front of the right.
- Slowly return to the starting position and perform the desired number of repetitions before completing on the opposite side.

Modifications

You can also perform this exercise with an explosive switching of the feet similar to the split jerk instead of the step-through described here. This would be considered a slight progression.

Tips

- Try performing this exercise with and without the coil position that involves throwing the elbow. You will likely feel significantly more speed and power with the elbow-through because of the role the lats play in rotational power.
- As you get more comfortable with this move and progress in loads, picture yourself winding up slightly and then exploding to uncoil and maximize power in this exercise.

PUSH PRESS

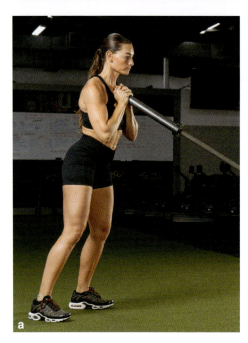

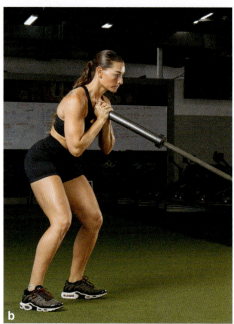

Muscles Targeted

This exercise, like the two-arm press, targets the shoulders, triceps, and upper chest and adds an element of power development from the posterior chain.

Starting Position

Stand facing the end of the barbell with the feet slightly wider than hip width and hands securely cradling the far end of the barbell with fingers interlaced. Body should be fully locked out and leaned forward into the bar with more weight on the balls of the feet. Elbows should be tight against the ribs and hands right against the sternum (a).

Coaching Cues

- Simultaneously bend the hips and knees to slightly lower the body and load the hips (b).

- Maintain core stiffness and explode upward, initiating the movement with the lower body to extend the hips and knees.

- As the weight drives upward and outward, finish the movement by also locking out the arms centered in front of the body *(c)*.
- Maintain stiffness at the top of the exercise to control momentum, and then lower back down in a controlled manner to the starting position.

Modifications

The push press is a great way to introduce power to your training and can also be performed from the full kneeling position, as well as the staggered stance included in this chapter.

Tips

- Make sure you have spent some time developing a foundation of strength in each of the foundational pressing positions before adding the push-press variation to any of them.
- You will also find that with the drop of the hips involved, you may need to maintain a slightly more forward lean into the bar for good alignment.

SPLIT JERK

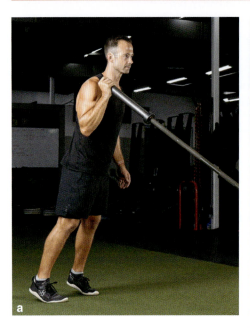
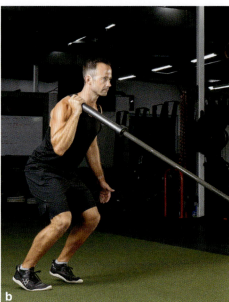

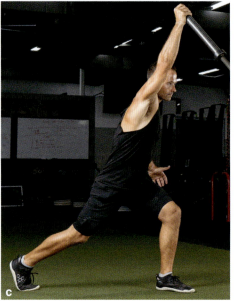

Muscles Targeted

This exercise targets the entire body but is mostly driven by the glutes, core, and shoulders.

Starting Position

Hold the landmine securely at the far end with the right hand near the shoulder and elbow held tight to the body. Feet are hip width and facing forward toward the landmine anchor *(a)*.

Coaching Cues

• Maintain a tight core position before executing the exercise.

• Slightly bend the hips and knees to dip down and load the body *(b)*.

• Powerfully drive up through the feet to push the landmine up and overhead while dropping down into a split-stance position with the right leg back to catch the weight *(c)*.

Modifications

You can also perform this exercise without finishing in the split position and just slightly dropping in to catch the weight overhead. This would be somewhat like the push press but without the split-stance landing component.

Tips

• This can be a great one for building full body stability in the catch position, so strive to get tight and stick the landing position before going for personal records with the overall load.

LATERAL SNATCH

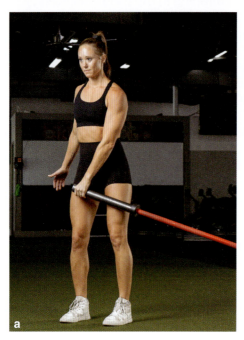
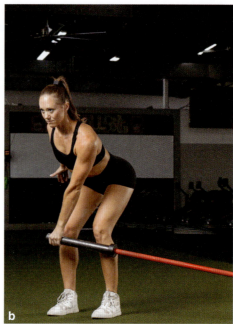

Muscles Targeted

This exercise targets the entire body but is mostly driven by the glutes, hamstrings, and shoulders.

Starting Position

Hold the landmine securely at the far end with the left hand just inside of the right thigh in front of the body. Feet are hip width or slightly wider with the toes pointed forward (a).

Coaching Cues

- Maintain a soft bend in the knees and hinge back at the hips to lower the landmine just below the knees (b).

- Tense the core while driving up and inward through the right foot so the landmine explodes up and to the left in a locked-out position and the left foot steps in toward the landmine (c).

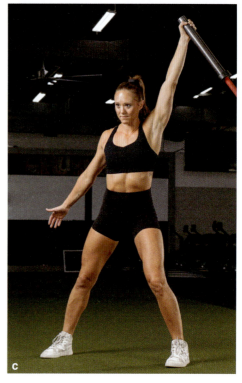

Modifications

This exercise can also be executed by landing into a split-stance position similar to the split jerk. Starting stance would be the same, but instead of stepping inward toward the landmine anchor when exploding up with the bar, the inside leg would end up back to catch the weight at the top in a split stance.

Tips

- This one is easy to try and muscle with the upper body, but when done right it should feel like it just flies up into position.
- Rather than driving the exercise with the arms, think about them as a string attached that just helps to guide it up and catch in the right position. This will make sure you are driving force through the legs and will likely limit the weights you can use with this power exercise.

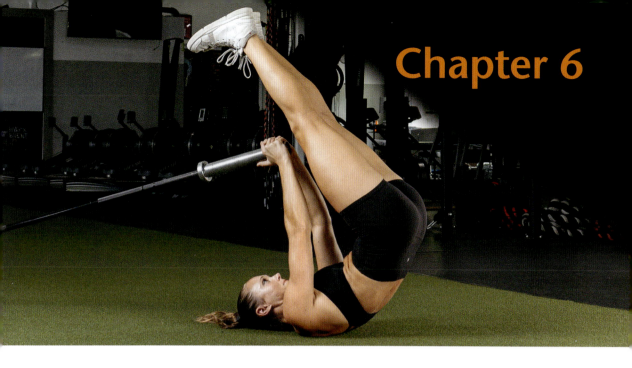

Chapter 6

CORE EXERCISES

This chapter includes landmine exercises geared toward building stability, strength, and power in the main core muscles that attach to the pelvis and spine. Most of the exercises involve a fair amount of full body engagement in using the landmine as a training tool but maintain a focus on the targeted core muscles.

The exercises in this chapter are ordered strategically to represent the skill level or difficulty associated with each exercise. This doesn't mean they aren't scalable to strength levels, but the ones that come earlier in the chapter will be easier to master. Make an effort to build upon these exercises by getting experience with them in the order in which they are listed and you'll be better set up for success.

SAFETY NOTE

Training with the landmine can be an effective way to strengthen the muscles of the hips and torso that help to both control and protect the low back. Some exercisers may not be as experienced with standing rotational exercises, so start all core exercises unloaded and master the technique before rushing to load with more weight or speed.

LANDMINE MARCH

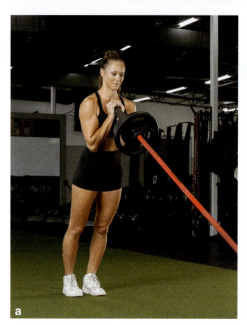 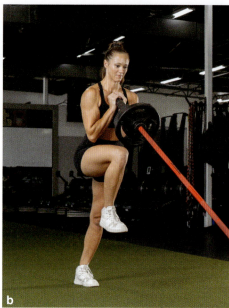

Muscles Targeted

This exercise targets all of the major muscles of the core.

Starting Position

Grip the far end of the barbell with hands interlaced and barbell held tight to the chest. Keep the feet close together stacked underneath the hips with a slight forward lean of the body into the bar *(a)*.

Coaching Cues

- Brace the core and squeeze the bar tight to the body to engage the muscles of the pecs and lats before initiating the movement.
- Slowly lift the right leg and knee up to a high-march position and pause for a second to ensure control *(b)*.
- Return slowly to the starting position and perform the same movement with the left leg for the desired reps or time. Keep the barbell in place at the chest, similar to the position for a weighted carry.

Modifications

Landmine marches serve as the foundation for other marching positions with the landmine, such as overhead marches. The overhead march is performed with nearly identical technique but the bar remains locked out overhead *(c)*, making it much more challenging to maintain balance and control. For added balance challenge, keep the rear foot elevated through the overhead lift phase *(d)*.

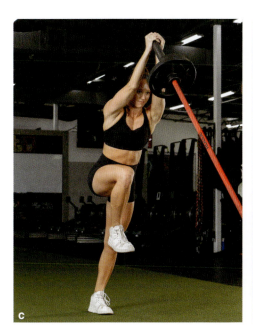 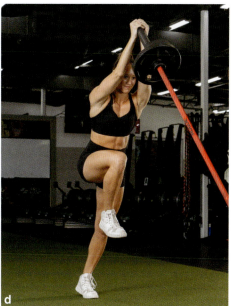

Tips

- Move slowly as you fine-tune your position because moving just slightly off of the midline will make it nearly impossible to maintain the landmine and torso position.

- This is a core stability exercise and is best performed with moderate loads for most exercisers to emphasize core and full body control.

LANDMINE ANCHORED DEADBUG

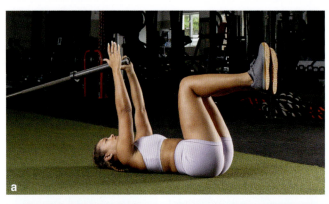

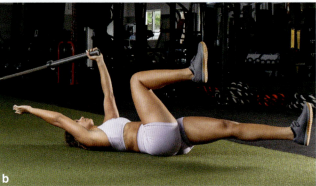

Muscles Targeted

This exercise targets all of the major core stabilizers but primarily hits the rectus abdominis and transverse abdominis.

Starting Position

Lie on your back facing away from the landmine anchor with your hips, knees, and ankles all bent to around 90 degrees so your low back is in contact with the ground and feet are in the air. Hold the very end of the barbell locked out in your left hand and elevated just in line with the shoulder and your right hand also locked out in line with the shoulder (a).

Coaching Cues

- Slowly extend your left leg out away from the body while simultaneously lowering the right arm toward the ground (b).
- Maintain core engagement so that the lower back doesn't come up much off the ground and exhale deeply as you return both the arm and leg back to the starting position.
- Complete all reps on one side, then change hands to repeat on the opposite side.

Modifications

This exercise could also be slightly regressed by placing both hands on the landmine and just focusing on the lower body portion of the movement *(c)*.

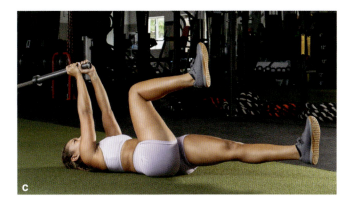

Tips

- Maintain stiffness and tightness in the arm holding the landmine to maximize core tension throughout the movement.
- Do your best to exhale fully on the way back in during each rep to maximize core contraction and prevent excessive breath holding.

LANDMINE ANCHORED REVERSE CRUNCH

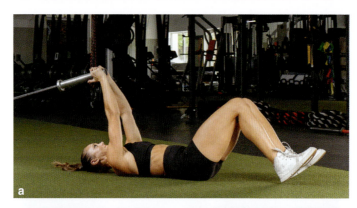

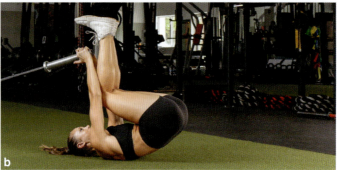

Muscles Targeted

This exercise primarily targets the rectus abdominis and hip flexors.

Starting Position

Lie on your back facing away from the landmine anchor with your low back and heels in contact with the floor and both knees and ankles bent to around 90 degrees. Hold the very end of the barbell locked out in both hands with one hand stacked over the other in line with the shoulders *(a)*.

Coaching Cues

- Firmly press the hands up into the landmine to use it as an anchor in initiating the exercise.
- Maintain the same bend in your knees and fully exhale as you curl your hips and lower body up toward the landmine so that the knees contact the elbows *(b)*.
- Slowly control one vertebra at a time back down to the starting position.

Modifications

This exercise could be intensified by straightening the legs to increase the load on the core *(c, d)*.

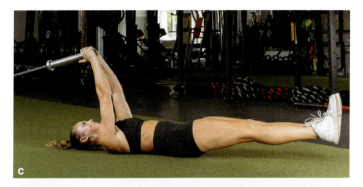

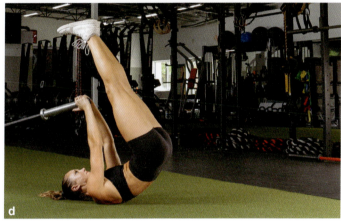

Tips

- Focus on slow control during the lowering phase back to the ground to maintain focus on the appropriate core muscles.

LANDMINE ANCHORED LEG LIFT

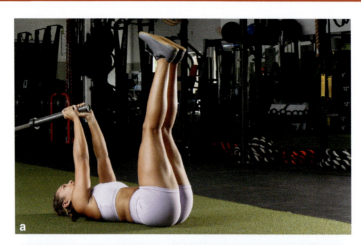

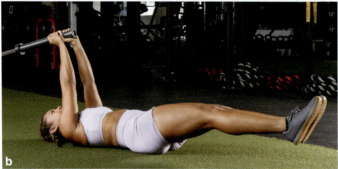

Muscles Targeted

This exercise primarily targets the rectus abdominis and hip flexors.

Starting Position

Lie on your back facing away from the landmine anchor with your legs held straight up into the air so that your low back is in contact with the ground. Keep your legs straight, if possible, otherwise a slight bend in the knees is OK. Hold the very end of the barbell locked out in both hands directly above the shoulders *(a)*.

Coaching Cues

- Drive both hands up into the landmine to create tension before starting the exercise.
- While maintaining low back contact with the ground, slowly lower your legs toward the ground until just before they touch *(b)*.
- Maintain core engagement so that the low back doesn't come up much off of the ground and exhale deeply as you return the legs to the starting position.

Modifications

This exercise could also be slightly regressed by only lowering one leg at a time from the top as it will be easier to manage the weight of just one leg while the other leg stays to minimize movement of the pelvis *(c)*. If this is too difficult, then regress to the deadbug.

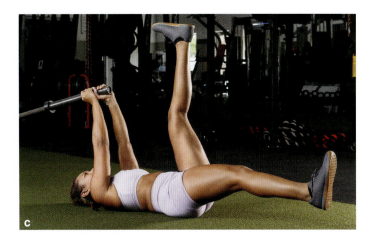

Tips

• Focus on slow controlled tempos and your breathing during the up and downward phases of the lift to ensure optimal core engagement.

LANDMINE STRAIGHT-LEG SIT-UP

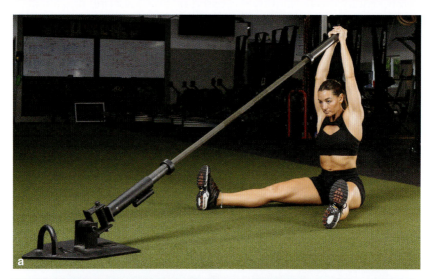

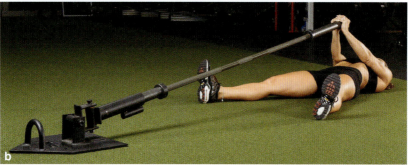

Muscles Targeted

This exercise primarily targets the rectus abdominis.

Starting Position

Take a tall seated stance on the ground with the landmine held locked out overhead with both hands. Legs should be straight and spread about 30 to 45 degrees with the barbell in line with the center of your body *(a)*.

Coaching Cues

- Brace the core and keep the arms as straight as possible.
- Slowly lower your body down to the floor by rolling down one vertebra at a time until you are lying fully on your back *(b)*.
- Maintain contact between your legs and the floor and exhale fully while you drive the bar back up to your starting position.
- While at the bottom in between reps, feel free to maintain a natural neutral curvature of the spine.

Modifications

If needed, you could bend the arms at the bottom position and then press them up and out to give yourself a little bit of momentum on the way up *(c)*. This may be helpful for smaller exercisers who struggle with the unloaded weight of the landmine.

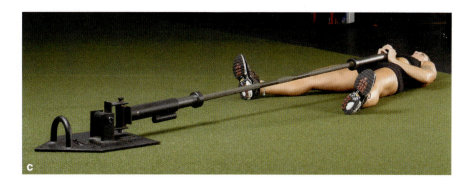

Tips

• Fight the urge to start from the bottom because you will end up spending more time trying to find your ideal position instead of just starting from the perfect top position.

• Also, do your best to avoid collapsing to the ground too fast and losing control.

TICKTOCKS

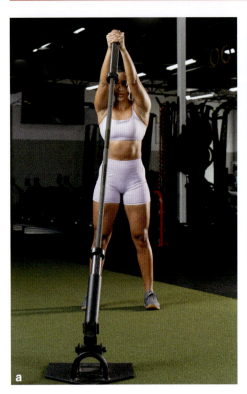

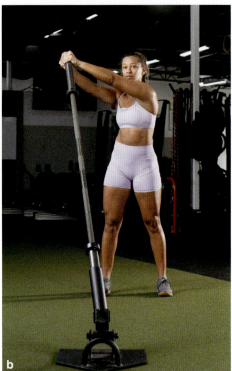

Muscles Targeted

This exercise targets most of the major muscles of the core but most specifically hits the obliques.

Starting Position

Stand with your feet slightly wider than hip width and face the landmine anchor. Grip the landmine with both hands interlaced and lock the arms out fully overhead in front of the body (a).

Coaching Cues

- Create some tension and brace the core before the movement to maintain stability and stiffness.
- Slowly rotate to the right to allow the bar to travel about 12 inches (30.5 cm) and then create tension to slow it down and reverse the direction (b).

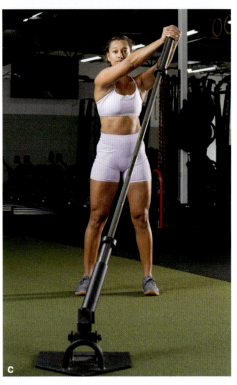

- Bring the bar back across the center of the body and without pausing, repeat the movement to the left side *(c)*, allowing the bar to swing back and forth from side to side like a clock pendulum but traveling no farther than about 12 inches (30.5 cm) on either side of the center.

Modifications

This drill could also be performed from the full- and half-kneeling positions with the same upper body technique.

Tips

- Keep your range of motion small with this exercise; it's meant to help train your core to control the rotation and side-to-side movement of the landmine.

OFFSET CORE ROTATIONS

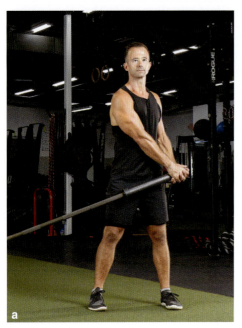
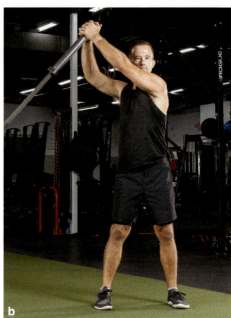

Muscles Targeted

This exercises the obliques as well as major muscles of the low back.

Starting Position

Stand with your feet slightly wider than hip width with your body parallel to the barbell so that it sticks out slightly beyond the left side of the body. Grip the barbell at the very end with an underhand grip on the left side and an overhand grip on the right and a relatively stiff straight arm position *(a)*.

Coaching Cues

- Brace the core and ensure the arms are stiff before initiating the exercise.
- Rotate through the core to bring the barbell up and out to the right side until the landmine is overhead and exactly parallel with the line of your body *(b)*.
- Pause at the top for control and then control slowly down to the start position in the same arc path.

Modifications

The more the arms are bent in this exercise, the less torque it will place on the core (easier it will feel), so bend the arms slightly if needed with higher relative loads. This movement could also be performed with a little bit of rotation in the back foot to make it slightly more athletic or to begin introducing rotational power *(c)*.

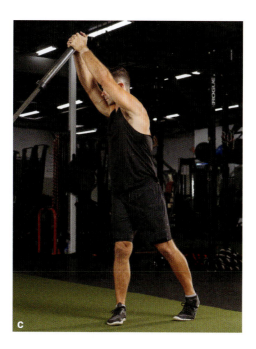

Tips

- Play with your position relative to the bar and width of your stance to find your strongest position.
- Maintain a slight soft bend in the knees and hips to minimize low back strain and make sure the muscles of the hips are helping to stabilize your body during this exercise.

RAINBOWS

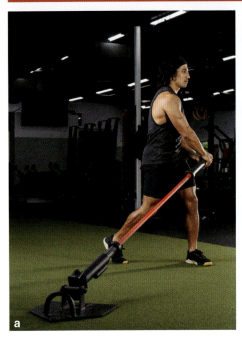

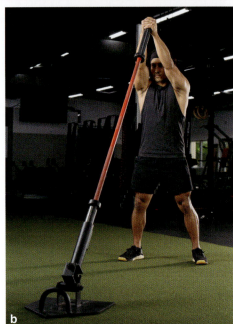

Muscles Targeted

This exercise targets most of the major muscles of the core, including the glutes, but primarily targets the obliques.

Starting Position

Stand with your feet slightly wider than hip width rotated just slightly left of the landline anchor point. Grip the landmine with both hands interlaced and maintain a bend in both arms just outside of the left hip *(a)*.

Coaching Cues

- Squeeze your hands on the bar to create stiffness in the upper body and brace the core before the movement.

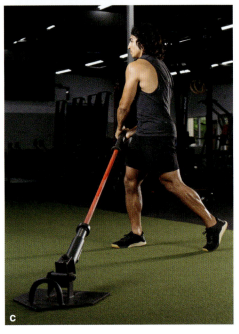

- Push through the left to rotate the body to the right and bring the bar up and across to the center of the body in line with the landmine anchor *(b)*.

- Without pausing in the middle, continue to rotate the feet and hips to the right to control the barbell down to just outside of the right side of the body *(c)*.

Modifications

Once mastered with control and adequate core strength, this movement can also be performed with more explosive tempos for rotational power training.

Tips

• Your stance should feel athletic, so make sure to rotate the feet and hips during this movement as well as maintain a soft bend in both the knees and elbows.

TALL KNEELING OFFSET ROTATIONS

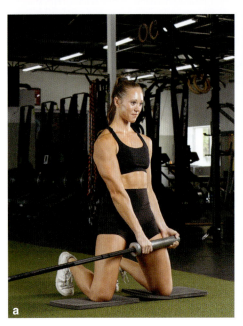 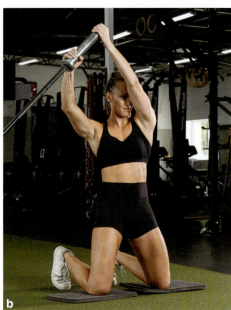

Muscles Targeted

This exercises the obliques as well as major muscles of the low back.

Starting Position

Take a tall kneeling stance with knees just wider than hip width with your body parallel to the barbell so that it sticks out slightly beyond the left side of the body. Grip the barbell at the very end with an underhand grip on the left side and an overhand grip with the right and a relatively stiff straight arm position (a).

Coaching Cues

- Brace the core and ensure the arms are stiff before initiating the exercise.
- Rotate through the core to bring the barbell up and out to the right side until the landmine is overhead and exactly parallel with the line of your body (b).
- Pause at the top for control and then control slowly down to the start position in the same arc path.

Modifications

The load of the barbell will be heavier in the kneeling position, so this movement could be modified back to the standing position with offset core rotations, as needed.

Tips

- Keep your toes dug into the ground and glutes squeezed to increase stability in your stance rather than allow for them to relax behind you.
- Maintaining tension in the glutes will help to maintain hip stability while you work to overcome the weight and rotate through the rest of your core and torso.

LANDMINE ROLLOUT

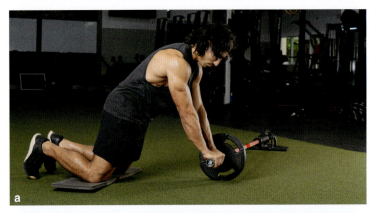

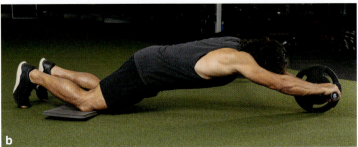

Muscles Targeted

This exercise targets all major muscles of the anterior core but specifically challenges the rectus abdominis, with some assistance from the lats.

Starting Position

Assume a full kneeling position perpendicular to the end of the landmine with knees slightly wider than hip width. Reach down with both hands to grip the far end of the barbell and maintain a slight "crunched" forward position (a).

Coaching Cues

- Dig your toes into the ground and maintain tension in the front of the core before initiating the exercise.
- Slowly roll the landmine out by only moving through the shoulders as far out as you can without losing torso position (b).
- Drive down through the landmine to keep the lats engaged and to bring the barbell back to the starting position.
- Repeat on the opposite side of the barbell.

Modifications

Using Olympic-style training plates will elevate the barbell higher off of the ground and make it easier to maintain optimal position in the hips and core *(c)*. If opting for this modification, don't use anything less than 25-pound training plates because the lighter ones may bend during the exercise.

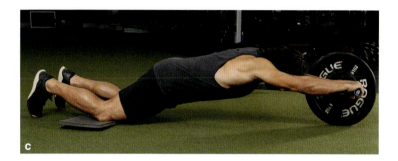

Tips

- Only go out as far as you can maintain your perfect starting position.
- Many will mistakenly allow the hips to move or the lower back and hips to cave, but the only thing that should truly move throughout the exercise is the shoulder joint while maintaining stiffness throughout the core.

BEAR POSITION TICKTOCK

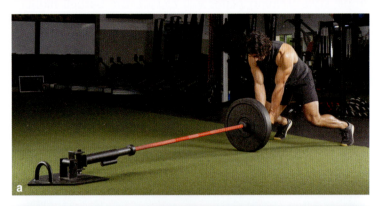

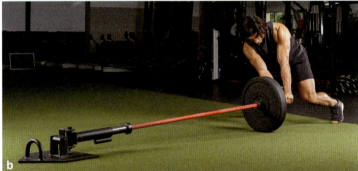

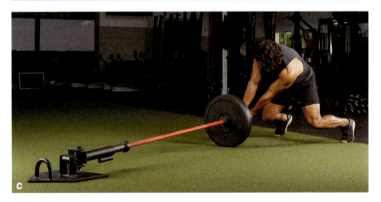

Muscles Targeted

This exercise targets the rectus abdominis and also brings in the obliques.

Starting Position

Face the end of the landmine so the barbell is in a straight line in front of the body. Assume a kneeling position with the knees above the ground and place one hand just above the other to grip the far end of the landmine with the hands in line with the chest. Push the shoulder blades apart, brace the core, and then bend the knees to around 90 degrees to achieve a flat back position *(a)*.

Coaching Cues

- Maintain the torso and hip position while slowly rolling the bar slightly out to the right of the body just off of the midline *(b)*.
- Brace the core and slightly rotate back to the left side to complete the same movement on the opposite side of the body *(c)*.
- Repeat this side-to-side motion slowly with no pause in the middle and change hand position from set to set.

Modifications

If this position is too challenging to hold, you can prop the knees up with a small plyometric box or pads to support the lower body during the exercise or just bring the knees to the ground *(d)*. A greater range of motion will also be much more demanding on the obliques and other muscles of the core.

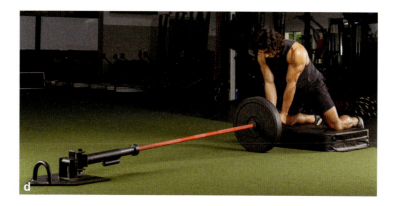

Tips

- Start with very small side-to-side movements before increasing the range of motion.
- You may also want to assume a wider position of the feet to give better leverage and stability during the exercise.

BEAR POSITION BODY SAW

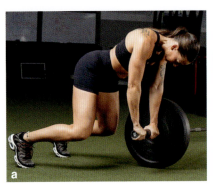
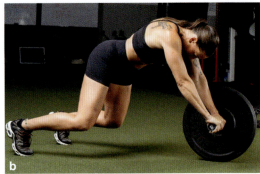

Muscles Targeted

This exercise targets the rectus abdominis and lats to stabilize the core.

Starting Position

Place your hands directly under the shoulders and grip the far end of the landmine with an overhand grip. Push the shoulder blades apart, brace the core, and then lift the knees off of the ground around 90 degrees to achieve a flat back position (a).

Coaching Cues

- Maintain torso and hip position while slowly rolling the bar slightly out in front of the body (b).
- Drive down through the bar and pull it back underneath the body to the starting position.
- Repeat the set on the opposite side of the bar.

Modifications

If this position is too challenging to hold, you can prop the knees up with a small plyometric box or pads to support the lower body during the exercise (c). Keep in mind that the range of motion can be increased or decreased to modify the intensity of the exercise.

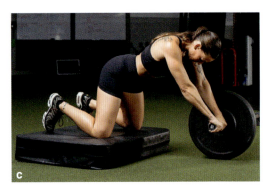

Tips

- Less is more with this exercise; it isn't meant to look like a rollout.
- Start slow with your arm movements and only roll out as far as you can maintain perfect body position for the desired reps.
- Which side of the landmine you're set up on won't make a massive difference here because the range of motion is small, but feel free to alternate sets on either side of the bar.

VARIATION: LANDMINE BEAR CRAWL

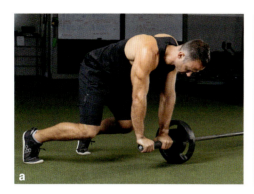
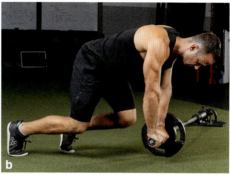

Muscles Targeted

All of them! This one could almost be considered full body, but it specifically targets the rectus abdominis and the internal and external obliques.

Starting Position

Place your hands directly under the shoulders and grip the far end of the landmine with an overhand grip. Push the shoulder blades apart, brace the core, and then bend the knees to around 90 degrees to achieve a flat back position (a).

Coaching Cues

- Maintain your weight over the top of the bar with your hands directly in line with the shoulders.
- Slowly take small "bear crawl" steps forward with the feet as far as the landmine can safely travel in one direction (b).
- Relax down and then repeat on the opposite side of the bar.

Modifications

To adjust the intensity of the exercise, you can use smaller or larger weight plates such as traditional 25-pound plates instead of the Olympic plates shown (c). You can also progress the exercise by not only crawling forward but also in reverse before switching sides of the landmine.

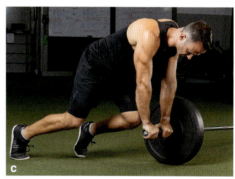

Tips

- If using smaller weight plates, avoid using anything less than a 25-pound plate, because smaller weights may fold and be unstable.
- Also, make sure you are using a home base–style or secure landmine base that will not tilt up with your weight on the far end.
- Go slow and take small steps during this exercise to maintain proper position.

VARIATION: WINDMILLS

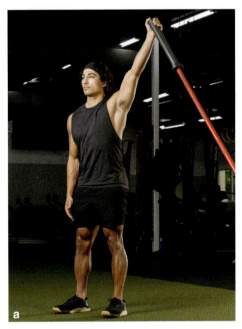 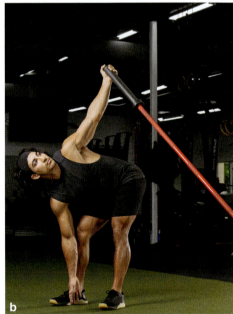

Muscles Targeted

The windmill could be considered a full body exercise, but with this landmine exercise we are focused on the obliques, quadratus lumborum, and glutes.

Starting Position

Stand perpendicular to the landmine with feet hip width. Grip the very end of the barbell with your left hand and arm locked out overhead *(a)*.

Coaching Cues

- Brace the core before initiating the movement.
- Maintain a soft bend in the knees as you simultaneously drive the hips back and to the left to lower your torso while keeping your eyes on the landmine in your left hand *(b)*.
- Pause for a second to ensure stability of the barbell and then slowly return to the starting position.

Modifications

To increase stability, you can press your nonworking arm into your outside leg as you slide down into the bottom position. This will help to create tension in the core and maintain a solid position as you are learning the exercise or managing heavier loads.

Tips

- This movement is great for improving core strength and stability at the hips and can serve as a great warm-up move on lower body days as well.
- Focus on slow tempos to maintain the focus on core control versus loading too heavy, too quickly.

BENT PRESS

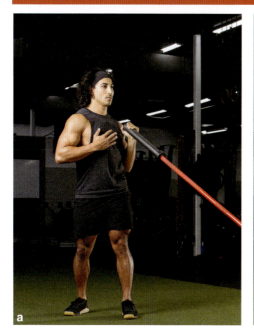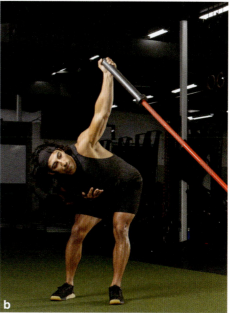

Muscles Targeted

The bent press is arguably a full body exercise, but with this landmine exercise we are focusing on the lateral muscles of the core, specifically the obliques and quadratus lumborum, with some assistance from the glutes.

Starting Position

Stand perpendicular to the landmine with feet hip width. Grip the very end of the barbell with your left hand at the shoulder and left elbow firmly against the ribs. Turn your shoulders just slightly to the left toward the landmine *(a)*.

Coaching Cues

- Brace the core before initiating the movement.
- Maintain a soft bend in the knees as you simultaneously drive the hips back and to the left while pressing the left arm up and out into a locked-out position *(b)*.
- Pause for a second to ensure stability of the barbell and then slowly return to your starting position.

Modifications

For those having any shoulder strain pressing in the position, opt for the windmill exercise also listed in this section.

Tips

- This one may take a few reps to fine-tune your distance to the bar, so warm-up with less load to better mark your position before loading.
- Also, minimize low back stress here by making sure to hinge back and to the side from the hips, similar to an RDL, rather than flexing laterally at the spine.

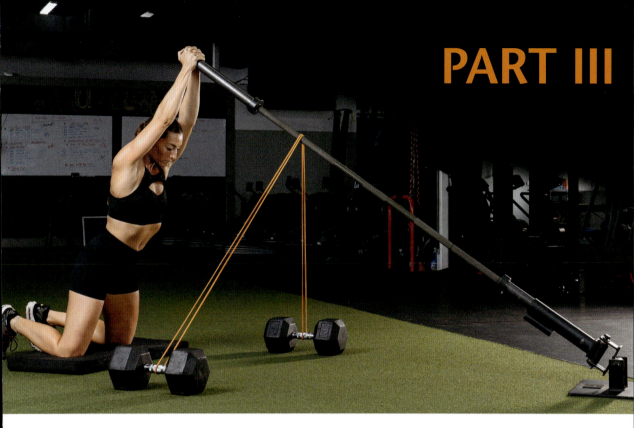

LANDMINE PROGRAMS

Part 3 shows you exactly how to maximize everything you have learned in parts 1 and 2 to develop complete landmine training programs. These sample workouts include examples of how to best integrate the landmine as a standalone training tool as well as a part of a complete program using other equipment.

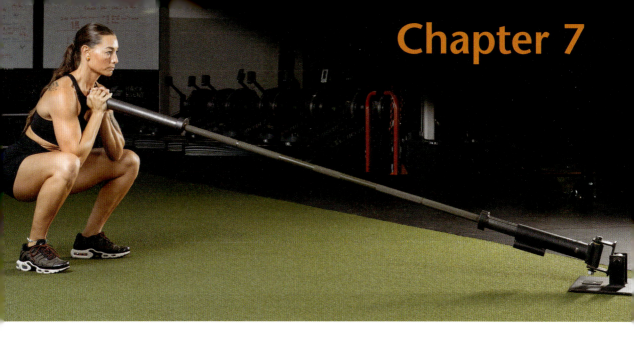

FOUNDATIONS OF PROGRAM DESIGN

Something is better than nothing when it comes to working out, but workouts with a hodgepodge of exercises will only get you so far. Long-term progress means having a plan that will allow you to continue to systematically overload the body.

However, this does not mean that your workout routine needs to be dull and inflexible. There is plenty of room for fun and variety, but to achieve optimal results, a relatively systematic approach is required in terms of exercise selection, progression, and overload. In this chapter, we dive into the foundational principles and variables that form the basis of the programs included in this book. These principles should guide your decision-making process at the gym and help you achieve your desired fitness goals.

BASIC PRINCIPLES

When creating a training program, it is important to take into account six key principles that form the foundation for effective training. These principles are progressive overload, load variation, specificity, individuality, diminishing returns, and reversibility. By addressing each of these principles, you can maximize your progress and ensure that your improvements are sustainable over time.

Progressive Overload

The human body naturally strives to maintain balance, or homeostasis, by adapting to both internal and environmental stressors. Exercise is a form of stress on the body, and to see physical changes, we must gradually and consistently increase the level of stress placed on the body. This gradual increase is known as progressive overload.

To achieve long-term progress, it is essential to manage the amount of stress placed on the body over time, finding the ideal balance. If the stress or frequency of training is not enough, we may not see progress. However, if we push ourselves too hard or too frequently for extended periods, we may risk injury.

Effective training requires finding the balance between challenging the body enough to drive adaptation, while also allowing adequate rest and recovery.

Load Variation

Driving progress in the body involves progressively introducing a greater level of stress, but this does not necessarily mean always lifting heavier weights or training harder. This strict linear approach may work initially, but, eventually, the body needs time to recover to see continued physical gains. This is where the concept of periodization comes into play.

Periodization involves strategically managing stress over time by incorporating phases into the training program where intensity and volume may be reduced to allow for adaptation. These short-term fluctuations and training weeks with less load help to maintain longer-term fitness gains throughout the year.

By varying loads, we can maximize our progress and minimize the risk of injury or burnout. This approach allows the body to recover and adapt, leading to sustained improvements in physical fitness over time.

Specificity

The principle of specificity in training dictates that we will see the greatest improvements in the areas we focus on. For instance, a training program designed to improve one's vertical jump will look very different from one designed to improve their 5K running time. To improve running performance, both running and strength training for muscular endurance are necessary because the two will complement each other. In contrast, improving vertical jump performance requires maximal strength and power training, with no running involved.

The principle of specificity can be applied in many ways, such as emphasizing particular types of muscle contractions, speed of movement, energy systems involved, and the mechanics of the exercise. Every exercise doesn't need to look identical to the quality or skill being trained, but it should target and improve the underlying systems that contribute to the overall goal.

Individuality

Although humans have similar physiological characteristics, the response to training programs can vary considerably among individuals due to factors such as genetics, fitness level, and limb lever length. It is tempting to follow the workout program of celebrities like Ryan Reynolds, but such programs may not be suitable for beginners, and they could lead to overtraining.

The choice of exercise technique and types of exercises can differ significantly among individuals with shorter or longer limbs. For instance, the biomechanics of the squat may vary considerably based on leg length, and the level of activation of the quadriceps and glutes may differ. Similarly, the mechanics of the bench press can vary depending on the individual's arm length, which can affect the activation of the chest and triceps muscles.

The training program can have a significant effect on muscle mass, strength, and power; however, genetic factors may also play a role in determining an individual's response to training. For example, some individuals may be more genetically inclined to respond favorably to lower reps and heavier loads when building muscle, whereas others may benefit more from higher-volume training.

Diminishing Returns

The longer and more consistently you train, the harder results are to come by. Beginner exercisers can do nearly anything for 8 to 12 weeks and see progress, but over time the rate of improvement slows. The concept of diminishing returns refers to the idea that as an individual becomes stronger, the rate of their strength gains decreases over time. For example, a beginner lifter may be able to increase their squat by 20 pounds (9 kg) within a month of training, but an advanced lifter may only be able to increase their squat by 5 pounds (2.3 kg) in the same time frame.

This is due to a variety of factors, including genetics, training history, and age, all of which contribute to the individual's ability to make progress.

As a result, strength training programs often incorporate periodization and other techniques to help individuals continue making gains, even as they reach a point of diminishing returns. The landmine can be a powerful tool for battling this concept because of the novel stimulus it provides across a spectrum of training goals and where it lives along the stability continuum.

Reversibility

The reversibility principle of exercise, commonly referred to as the "use it or lose it" principle, implies that the benefits of training can gradually diminish or be lost entirely when an individual discontinues or reduces the intensity or frequency of their exercise routine. In simpler terms, the gains in strength, endurance, flexibility, and other fitness components can slowly fade over time if a person stops training them.

This book outlines the power of the landmine as a unique tool for training antirotation, force transfer, and full body stability, as discussed in chapter 1. However, it is essential to note that if certain aspects of these abilities are not incorporated into the training program using the landmine or other equipment, the body will regress in these skills.

TRAINING VARIABLES

The previous section was about the overarching principles that should guide a training program, but this section gets into the specific variables involved in designing your sessions. This should include the careful consideration of frequency, intensity, volume, tempo, and rest. Your decisions regarding each of these variables should be tied directly to your training goals, but they may also be affected by your desired training frequency and what kind of training experience you enjoy.

Frequency

The frequency of training is the number of workout sessions performed within a given week. The ideal training frequency is highly dependent on various factors, such as training experience, time commitments, preferences, and goals. For individuals seeking general fitness and health improvements, a training frequency of two to three sessions a week is often sufficient.

However, more ambitious goals such as building muscle mass may require a higher frequency of three to six sessions per week. It's important to note that while increasing the number of training sessions may seem like a straightforward approach to achieving your fitness goals, it's not always the right answer.

It's essential to find a balance between training frequency and allowing sufficient recovery time for the body. Overtraining can result in fatigue, injury, and decreased performance. Additionally, it's crucial to consider the intensity and duration of each training session to avoid burnout and ensure consistency.

Intensity

In the realm of fitness, the term *intensity* has multiple meanings, but when it comes to training, it is commonly referred to as the training load, which is the weight used during an exercise. It is also regarded as one of the most crucial factors in determining the results of a training program or training block.

If you aim to increase muscular endurance, you should opt for loads that you can handle for at least 12 to 20 repetitions or more. However, if your goal is to maximize strength gains and improve force output, you should use heavier loads that you can only complete six repetitions or fewer with.

When it comes to hypertrophy and muscle gain, research has shown that a variety of rep ranges can be effective as long as the weight and repetition scheme allows you to reach true mechanical failure (Schoenfeld et al. 2017). This finding highlights the importance of selecting exercises from this book that allow you to train at the appropriate intensities to achieve your desired results.

Volume

Volume is the total amount of work done during a single training session, which includes the number of sets, reps, and exercises performed. For example, if someone performs three sets of 10 reps of squats, they have completed a volume of 30 reps for that exercise. Similarly, if they perform four different exercises in their workout session, the total volume of training would be the sum of all the sets, reps, and exercises performed. Increasing the volume of training over time can help to stimulate muscle growth and improve overall fitness levels. However, it is important to gradually increase the volume of training to avoid overtraining and injury.

Tempo

Tempo is one of the most crucial but often neglected training variables. Most people focus on sets, reps, and weights, overlooking the impact of their movement speed. This is a mistake and can leave gains on the table. For example, if you go too fast when you're trying to build muscle, you may rely more on momentum and place less demand on the muscles. Applying appropriate tempos during exercises can significantly improve training outcomes at all levels. For instance, for overall fitness and muscular endurance, using slower eccentrics and purposeful isometrics can significantly enhance motor control and stability.

Speeding Through Reps

Speeding through a rep can lead to performing the exercise improperly, engaging the wrong muscles, or relying on momentum instead of muscles to complete the movement. This improper execution not only diminishes the effectiveness of the exercise but also increases the risk of injury. When the tempo is too fast, it becomes challenging to maintain proper form and control, making it easier to lose balance or strain muscles and joints inappropriately.

Research on Tempo

Research shows that manipulating tempo can have distinct impacts on muscle hypertrophy and strength development. A study by Schoenfeld et al. (2015) found that slower tempos, especially during the eccentric (lowering) phase, can lead to greater muscle damage and hypertrophy due to increased time under tension. Another study by Hatfield et al. (2006) indicated that varying tempo can influence neural adaptations and muscle recruitment patterns, optimizing strength gains.

Pinpointing the Right Training Tempo

To determine the right tempo for your training goals, consider the following guidelines:

- *Endurance and control.* Opt for a slower tempo like 4-2-2-2 (4 seconds lowering, 2 seconds pause, 2 seconds lifting, 2 seconds pause) to improve muscular endurance, control, and stability.
- *Muscle hypertrophy.* Use a moderate tempo such as 3-1-2-1 (3 seconds lowering, 1 second pause, 2 seconds lifting, 1 second pause). This allows for increased time under tension, which is essential for muscle growth.
- *Strength.* Implement a tempo of 2-0-X-0 (2 seconds lowering, no pause, explosive concentric phase, no pause) to focus on maximal muscle recruitment and neural adaptations.
- *Power.* For power training, employ a faster tempo of 1-0-X-0 (1 second lowering, no pause, explosive concentric phase, no pause) to enhance explosive strength and speed.

By manipulating the tempo of an exercise, we can also add intensity and variety without increasing the overall training load. This can be a safer and more suitable method of progression for some exercises. Pay attention to the tempos described in each of the following chapters to ensure you are approaching the exercises in each program with the appropriate training tempos.

Rest

Rest is an essential factor that plays a vital role in between sets and training sessions. The rest duration has a significant impact on the quality of the workout and its results. Rest too little and you could be underperforming, but rest too long and you could be wasting time at the gym.

To enhance muscular endurance, it is recommended to have rest periods of 30 to 60 seconds between sets of the same muscle or muscle groups. To increase muscular fitness or muscle size, a rest period of 30 to 90 seconds between sets is sufficient. However, if you alternate between opposing muscle groups, such as the biceps and triceps or lower body and upper body exercises, you may not need as long. Super setting in this way—performing one exercise and then resting only 20 to 30 seconds before performing the next—can provide sufficient rest between muscle groups and still allow for optimal performance. This can be an extremely engaging and time-efficient way for many exercisers to train.

For those aiming to gain higher levels of strength and power, it is crucial to have more extended rest periods ranging from two to five minutes. This ensures that energy stores are fully replenished and there is sufficient effort for subsequent repetitions.

It is equally important to consider the rest required between training sessions. To allow sufficient recovery, a minimum of 48 hours is recommended for a consistent training program between training sessions of the same muscle group or movement.

See table 7.1 for basic recommendations on each training variable when building programs around a specific goal set.

This chapter has introduced some of the main concepts that come together to create a great training program, and while many of them require extensive experience and study to master, the next best step is to experience them in action. In the following chapters, we will delve into specific training plans that utilize these principles to optimize your landmine training. These plans are designed to help you systematically progress, ensuring you continue to challenge your body while allowing for adequate recovery and adaptation. By following these structured programs, you can maximize your gains, minimize the risk of injury, and keep your workouts engaging and effective.

Let's move forward and explore the detailed training plans that will guide you to your fitness goals with precision and purpose.

Table 7.1   Basic Training Guidelines

	Frequency	Intensity	Volume	Speed (tempo)	Rest
Muscular endurance	2-3 ×/week	60% of 1RM	• 1 or 2 exercises per muscle group or movement • 2 or 3 sets for each muscle group or movement • 10-20 reps of each exercise	Variable	30-60 sec between muscle groups
Muscular fitness	3-4 ×/week	60-75% of 1RM	• 1 or 2 exercises per muscle group or movement • 3-6 sets for each muscle group or movement • 10-12 reps of each exercise	Moderate	30-90 sec between muscle groups
Muscle size	3-6 ×/week	60-75% of 1RM	• 2 or 3 exercises per muscle group or movement • 3-6 sets for each muscle group or movement • 6-20 reps of each exercise	Slow to moderate	60-90 sec between muscle groups
Muscular strength	3-6 ×/week	Basic strength: 80-90% of 1RM	• 1-3 exercises per muscle group or movement • 4-8 reps	Slow	2-5 min between muscle groups
Muscular power	2-3 ×/week	75-90% for multiple reps Variable when body weight	• 1-6 reps per exercise • 6-10 reps for body weight–based power exercises	Fast	2-5 min between muscle groups

Adapted by permission from D. Wathen, T.R. Baechle, and R.W. Earle, "A Periodization Model for Resistance Training," in *Essentials of Strength Training and Conditioning,* 3rd ed., by the National Strength and Conditioning Association, edited by T.R. Baechle and R.W. Earle (Champaign, IL: Human Kinetics), 511.

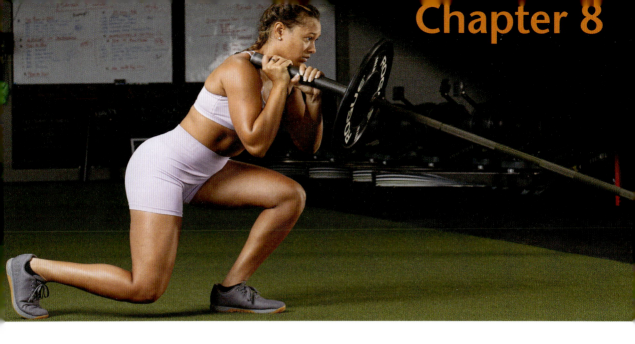

Chapter 8

TOTAL BODY CONDITIONING

Utilizing the landmine as a training tool goes beyond just achieving peak performance; it is also about promoting optimal health and longevity. We mentioned in chapter 1 that functional training is all about achieving physical freedom, and, if used effectively, the landmine can help you get more out of life. However, it all starts with building the right base of training.

Muscular and cardiorespiratory conditioning are likely crucial components of achieving this goal and form the basis for a holistic approach to fitness and training. Although these two aspects are often viewed as separate entities, the workouts in this chapter use the landmine as a resistance training tool to establish a foundation that benefits both.

Total body conditioning is often discussed as a method for developing overall muscular fitness, but the total body focus benefits the entire body system. It is ideal for laying a strong foundation for training technique, building muscular endurance, preventing injury, and bridging the gap between traditional strength and cardiovascular training.

BUILDING THE ICEBERG—TRAINING FOR LIFE

Muscular fitness may have a loosely defined meaning in training because it can imply improving endurance, size, strength, and power simultaneously. In this chapter, the concept of fitness is focused primarily on building a basis of muscular endurance and total body stability. This approach to training is also often referred to in exercise programming periodization as developing general physical preparedness (GPP), or a solid foundation of training to build off of after a period of less training intensity.

I'm not a fan of the term *GPP* for most people, because it doesn't always land and explain the focus. It also doesn't make a strong enough case for the fact that total body conditioning doesn't just have to be a starting point.

Total body conditioning may be one of the most effective and beneficial ways for a vast majority of people to train for a lifetime. So for the sake of better understanding our initial approach and some of the benefits of training this type of general muscular fitness, picture an iceberg like the one shown in figure 8.1.

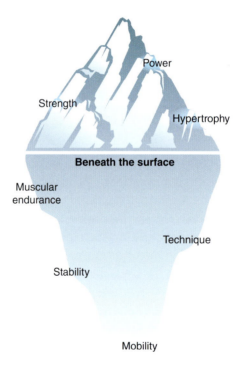

Figure 8.1 This figure represents various components of fitness and athleticism. The capacities above the surface are often what we focus on in our training programs, but their potential depends upon the base we have established with the components that lie below the surface.

Most people think about the results from resistance training as the "above the surface," visible and noticeable training outcomes, such as increases in muscle size, strength, and even explosiveness. You might think of these as some of the more aesthetic, athletic, or performance-based outcomes that strength training is well known for improving.

These outcomes are well documented and worth training for, but there are several less sexy "beneath the surface" qualities that most exercisers would greatly benefit from improving as they look to lay down a lifelong foundation for strength training. This is where taking the time to improve things like mobility, stability, and exercise-specific technique can pay massive dividends. As is often described in traditional GPP programs, it doesn't mean you won't also make some ancillary improvements in the "above the surface" qualities. Results for most will likely spill over into some muscle and strength gains, but the primary focus is on the variables in the image that often sit "below the surface."

As you will find in the following chapters, it's not about isolating specific exercises to just one phase of training or the other, but rather about how you put them together, the exercise skill level required, the variables used, and the intent put into every movement. This doesn't mean these total body conditioning workouts will by any means be easy (quite the opposite), but this first programming chapter should serve as a great starting point to building an iceberg that will stand the test of time.

IMPROVING MOVEMENT QUALITY

You can think of movement quality as exercise technique, but a more relevant definition for this book would be that it is the ability to efficiently execute an exercise with the full available range of motion. Specific flexibility and mobility training are beyond the scope of this book, but the most effective way we can use strength training to enhance these things is to prioritize training the greatest range of motion in every exercise possible over increased load.

Simply put, try to move well before stressing about moving heavy or fast. You will get the most out of these total body conditioning programs if you don't sacrifice perfect position or full range of motion for more weight or reps. Over time, this will pay big dividends in increasing stability and control at the end range of motion, where injuries are likely to occur with training.

Tempo is also one of the most underutilized tools for improving movement quality. You hear the word *conditioning* and might immediately think "fast-paced," but early in this phase of training we want the exact opposite. We want to minimize momentum and maximize control. One of the most effective ways to initially improve the quality of your movements is to slow everything down. As you progress to the power chapter in this book, you will see we don't believe in moving slowly forever, but it has value. Exercise is inherently a skill, and slowing things down will give you better practice, especially with some of the landmine exercises that demand more full body stability or coordination.

TOTAL BODY BENEFITS AND FREQUENCY

You'll find that there aren't a ton of isolation exercises in this book. This isn't because they don't have value, but rather because the landmine is far more of a full body training tool. Even most of the upper body, lower body, or core exercises involve a lot of engagement from the rest of the body. The landmine can be integrated into nearly any type of training split, but as a cornerstone or stand-alone tool it may be best utilized as a total body training piece. Total body training workouts offer some big advantages for a wide variety of exercisers, such as:

- *Training efficiency.* You can accomplish a lot of overall work in a short amount of time or with less frequency. This is helpful for people who don't have four to five days a week to train.
- *Increased frequency.* The increased frequency allows for training the same body parts two to three times a week to better build up tolerance for training and improve motor learning.
- *Maintained focus.* Total body workouts leave less time for isolation and excessive volume, which may actually detract from some fitness goals.

We recommend most people stick with a frequency of two to three times per week if just starting a total body conditioning program; more than that can be challenging to adequately recover from.

INCORPORATING LANDMINE TRAINING INTO A TOTAL BODY CONDITIONING PROGRAM

One of the reasons the landmine is such a powerful training tool is because of its versatility and ability to serve as a stand-alone corner gym. This means you can train the entire body without much equipment and in a relatively small footprint. This makes it an exceptionally effective stand-alone training tool, especially for total body training programs like those found in this chapter.

However, you will most often find the landmine as a cornerstone tool integrated into a bigger-picture program that mixes modalities and equipment. Some of the landmine exercises introduced in this book serve as upgrades or replacements to some traditional strength and power moves and are best suited to be plugged in at the appropriate place in a general total body program.

We have provided examples of each in the landmine training total body conditioning programs that follow. This means you can use some of them as additions to your current total body program or use them as a stand-alone strength training program.

Here are a few overarching key points regarding these workouts that will help you get the most out of them and adapt them as needed over time:

Rest

- The sets that follow in each workout are set up in either superset (A1, A2) or triplex (B1, B2, B3) fashion. This means they are meant to be done back to back with just enough rest between exercises to transition to the next move—ideally 20 to 40 seconds max. Once you have completed each one, you have completed an entire set and should take a full rest period.
- Rest for 60 to 90 seconds after completing an entire superset or triplex.

Reps/Time

- The priority here is the controlled and intentional execution of each rep with perfect technique.
- Minimize momentum and fight the urge to cheat reps to hit the rep range with a certain weight; instead, lower your weight as needed to hit the rep ranges included.
- Tempo matters here, so when in doubt slightly slow down the lowering phase (two to three seconds eccentric) and move normally with the lifting phase (one second concentric) of each exercise.

Intensity

- Leave a few reps in the tank on most of the exercises included in each workout for total body conditioning. It's good to challenge yourself with more load in this phase over time, but most sets you should finish knowing you probably still could have pushed out three or more good reps without compromising form. You will build muscular endurance and still likely gain some ancillary hypertrophy and strength without working to failure in this phase of training.
- If you measure your intensity on a scale from 0 to 10, with 10 representing total technique or muscular failure, then your goal should be to work up to just 7 or 8 on your final sets in each of the following workouts.

Substitute when necessary

- Great training programs are not about handcuffing you to exercises that aren't right for your body. If you find yourself in pain or uncomfortable with an exercise, don't force it.
- Chapter 7 talks about the concept of individuality, and we had this in mind when we built out the programming options that follow. We have included movement patterns in the workout programs that match the exercises listed in earlier chapters to give you programming options and the ability to adapt. Some moves may just not fit your body and how it

moves. Simply choose another exercise option in that movement category that you can perform through the full range of motion without pain.

LANDMINE-ONLY PROGRAM

This first training program is a total body conditioning template that could serve as a stand-alone approach toward strength training (see tables 8.1 and 8.2). For context, we define *lower body pushing* as exercises that are more knee dominant, such as squatting and lunging. *Lower body pulling* is defined as exercises that are more hip dominant and focus on the glutes, hamstrings, and low back. Pairing together total body workouts this way is not required, but it does have some additional benefits of allowing for low back, shoulder, and grip rest throughout each workout.

For your benefit in adapting some of the following programs, we have also included a movement column in each table that corresponds to the subcategories of push, pull, squat, lunge, hinge, full body, core, and accessory that are used to organize the exercises in chapters 3 through 6. This should enable you to easily make appropriate exercise substitutions (landmine exercises or not) when needed without having to change the overall programming. Any exercises not featured in this book will be denoted by "N/A" but can be easily looked up for better understanding.

These workouts could be completed as presented for an eight-week block by cycling back to week one after week four. Alternatively, you could progress to new movements after your first four-week block for some exercise variety or movement progression. For your convenience, we have also organized the exercises in each chapter and subcategory in relative order of progression to help you decide which exercise to tackle next.

Table 8.1 Total Body A (Lower Body Push, Upper Body Pull)

Exercise	Page	Movement	Week 1	Week 2	Week 3	Week 4
(A1) Top-loaded reverse lunge	102	Lunge	2 × 15/ side	3 × 12-15/ side	3 × 12/ side	4 × 10/ side
(A2) Meadows row	70	Pull	2 × 15/ side	3 × 12-15/ side	3 × 12/ side	4 × 10/ side
(B1) Landmine goblet squat	82	Squat	2 × 15	3 × 15	3 × 12-15	3 × 12
(B2) T-bar row (with towel)	66	Pull	2 × 15	3 × 15	3 × 12-15	3 × 12
(C1) Hack squat	88	Squat	2 × 15	3 × 15	3 × 15	3 × 12-15
(C2) Rainbows	188	Core	2 × 12/ side	3 × 12/ side	3 × 10/ side	3 × 8/ side
(C3) Landmine anchored leg lift	180	Core	2 × 10	3 × 10	3 × 12	3 × 15

Table 8.2 Total Body B (Lower Body Pull, Upper Body Push)

Exercise	Page	Movement	Week 1	Week 2	Week 3	Week 4
(A1) Staggered RDL	128	Hinge	2 × 15/ side	3 × 12-15/ side	3 × 12/ side	4 × 10/ side
(A2) Half-kneeling single-arm press	50	Push	2 × 15/ side	3 × 12-15/ side	3 × 12/ side	4 × 10/ side
(B1) Landmine sumo deadlift	136	Hinge	2 × 15	3 × 15	3 × 12-15	3 × 12
(B2) Single-arm floor press	60	Push	2 × 15/ side	3 × 15/ side	3 × 12-15/ side	3 × 12/ side
(C1) Kneeling push press (with hip extension)	150	Full body	2 × 15	3 × 15	3 × 15	3 × 12-15
(C2) Standing calf raise	138	Accessory	2 × 15	3 × 15	3 × 15	3 × 12-15
(C3) Landmine bear crawl	197	Core	2 × 1 min	3 × 1 min	3 × 1 min	3 × 1 min

LANDMINE ONLY:
FULL BODY WITH CORE EMPHASIS EXAMPLE

This workout (table 8.3) serves as one that could be tagged onto the program listed in tables 8.1 and 8.2 as a third training day in a given week or a stand-alone landmine session to be added to an existing weekly workout program.

It contains many of the same total body conditioning variables (reps, sets, etc.) but emphasizes landmine exercises that place an even greater demand on rotation and stability throughout the core.

Table 8.3   Landmine Only: Full Body With Core Emphasis Example

Exercise	Page	Movement	Week 1	Week 2	Week 3	Week 4
(A1) Tall kneeling offset rotations	190	Core	2 × 15/ side	2 × 12/ side	2 × 12/ side	3 × 10/ side
(A2) Landmine bear crawl	197	Core	2 × 30 sec	2 × 45 sec	2 × 60 sec	3 × 45 sec
(B1) Offset surfer squat	90	Squat	2 × 15/ side	3 × 12-15	3 × 12	4 × 10
(B2) Staggered single-arm row	68	Pull	2 × 15/ side	3 × 15/ side	3 × 12/ side	4 × 10/ side
(C1) Staggered single-arm press	44	Push	2 × 15/ side	3 × 15/ side	3 × 12-15/ side	3 × 12
(C2) Single-leg RDL	132	Hinge	2 × 15/ side	3 × 12-15/ side	3 × 12/ side	3 × 12/ side
(C3) Landmine anchored reverse crunch	178	Core	2 × 15	3 × 12	3 × 12	3 × 12

LANDMINE PLUS BODY WEIGHT EXAMPLE

The landmine workout in table 8.4 serves as a great example of how the landmine can also be a great tool to integrate into a total body conditioning program that also emphasizes body weight strength. This can be great for anyone working out with minimal equipment.

Table 8.4   Landmine Plus Body Weight Example

Exercise	Page	Movement	Week 1	Week 2	Week 3	Week 4
(A1) Elevated reverse lunge	106	Lunge	2 × 15/ side	3 × 15/ side	3 × 12/ side	4 × 10/ side
(A2) Pull-up (or TRX row)	N/A	Pull	2 × 15	3 × 12-15/ side	3 × 10-12	4 × 10-12
(A3) Standing two-arm landmine press	38	Push	2 × 15	3 × 15	3 × 12	4 × 10
(A4) Single-leg body weight bridge	N/A	Hinge	2 × 15/ side	3 × 12-15/ side	3 × 12-15/ side	4 × 12-15/ side
(C1) Adductor RDL	126	Hinge	2 × 15	3 × 15	3 × 12	4 × 10
(C2) Push-up variation	N/A	Push	2 × 15	3 × 12	3 × 10-12	4 × 10-12
(C1) Two-handed landmine row (prison row)	64	Pull	2 × 15	3 × 15	3 × 15	4 × 10/ side

GENERAL TOTAL BODY CONDITIONING

The program example that follows is the most likely way that the landmine will live on as part of most people's training programs. The landmine-only programs included in this book are brutally effective, but a well-rounded training program often takes advantage of multiple tools that are available to meet training goals and preferences.

The program in this section has been built around the movement categories already mentioned to allow for flexibility and uses commonly found gym equipment (cables, dumbbells, barbells, and the landmine). The three workouts in tables 8.5, 8.6, and 8.7 could be used for a three-day-a-week total body conditioning program; they could also be cycled through for a twice-a-week program for more weekly variety.

Table 8.5   Total Body A: General Conditioning

Exercise	Page	Movement	Week 1	Week 2	Week 3	Week 4
(A1) Dumbbell RDL	N/A	Hinge	2 × 15	3 × 15	3 × 12	4 × 12
(A2) Staggered single-arm press	44	Push	2 × 15/ side	3 × 15/ side	3 × 12/ side	4 × 10/ side
(B1) Angled Zercher reverse lunge	113	Lunge	2 × 15/ side	3 × 12-15/ side	3 × 12/ side	3 × 10/ side
(B2) Lat pull-down	N/A	Pull	2 × 15	3 × 15	3 × 12-15	3 × 12
(C1) Single-arm floor press	60	Push	2 × 15/ side	3 × 15/ side	3 × 12/ side	3 × 12/ side
(C2) Dumbbell walking lunges	N/A	Lunge	2 × 15/ side	3 × 12/ side	3 × 10/ side	3 × 8/side
(C3) Core cable chops	N/A	Core	2 × 15/ side	3 × 12/ side	3 × 12/ side	3 × 12/ side

Table 8.6 Total Body B: General Conditioning

Exercise	Page	Movement	Week 1	Week 2	Week 3	Week 4
(A1) Landmine goblet squat	82	Squat	2 × 15	3 × 15	3 × 12	4 × 12
(A2) Dumbbell bent-over row	N/A	Pull	2 × 15/ side	3 × 15/ side	3 × 12/ side	4 × 12/ side
(B1) Staggered RDL	128	Hinge	2 × 15/ side	3 × 12/ side	3 × 12/ side	3 × 12/ side
(B2) Dumbbell chest press	N/A	Push	2 × 15	3 × 15	3 × 12-15	3 × 12
(C1) Dumbbell lateral lunge	N/A	Lunge	2 × 15/ side	3 × 12/ side	3 × 10/ side	3 × 10/ side
(C2) Cable triceps extensions	N/A	Accessory	2 × 15	3 × 15	3 × 15	3 × 12-15
(C3) Ticktocks	184	Core	2 × 15/ side	3 × 12/ side	3 × 12/ side	3 × 12/ side

Table 8.7 Total Body C: General Conditioning

Exercise	Page	Movement	Week 1	Week 2	Week 3	Week 4
(A1) Rotational RDL-to-press	162	Full body	2 × 12/ side	2 × 12/ side	2 × 12/ side	3 × 10/ side
(A2) Lateral plank variation	N/A	Core	2 × 30 sec	2 × 45 sec	2 × 60 sec	3 × 30 sec
(B1) Bottom-loaded reverse lunge	108	Lunge	2 × 15/ side	3 × 12/ side	3 × 12/ side	4 × 10/ side
(B2) Dumbbell incline chest press	N/A	Push	2 × 15	3 × 15	3 × 12	4 × 12
(C1) Hack squat	88	Squat	2 × 15/ side	3 × 15	3 × 15	3 × 15
(C2) Single-arm high-cable row	N/A	Pull	2 × 15/ side	3 × 15/ side	3 × 12/ side	3 × 12/ side
(C3) Dumbbell hammer curl	N/A	Accessory	2 × 15	3 × 15	3 × 12	3 × 12

The landmine is an incredibly versatile and powerful tool for total body conditioning, offering benefits that extend far beyond traditional training methods. Even though many exercisers will be unlikely to only train with the landmine forever, committing to the landmine-only programs for a period of time can be a great way to master many of the movements in this book in the context of a well-organized program.

As you move forward, remember that the effectiveness of your training depends not only on the exercises you choose and how you pair them, but also on the intention and control you bring to each movement. If you don't compromise and you follow the principles and priorities laid out in this chapter, you will only continue to build more potential with the "above the surface" training goals that follow.

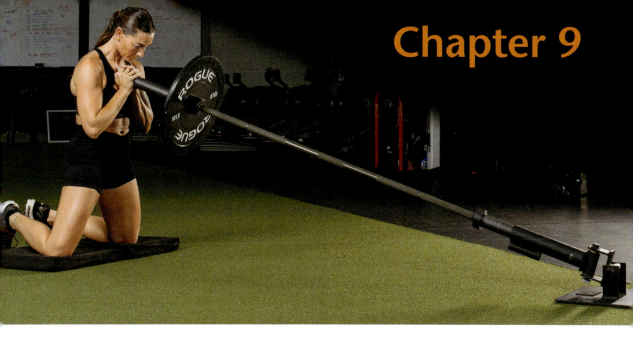

Chapter 9

ADVANCED CONDITIONING

Total body training programs like those in chapter 8 are not only one of the best ways to establish a rock-solid foundation of overall fitness, but, when programmed effectively they can also be extremely effective for fat loss and improving work capacity. The workouts in this chapter can be seen as a progression from the training programs found in chapter 8—hence, the term *advanced conditioning*. These workouts are for those who have already established proper technique, stability, and muscular endurance with the landmine as a tool.

MIXED-MODE TRAINING

Also commonly called a hybrid training approach, mixed-mode training purposely combines multiple training modalities into a single workout, such as strength training, cardiovascular routines, and plyometric exercises. The goal of mixed-mode training is to develop well-rounded fitness by targeting multiple fitness components simultaneously. It aims to improve overall physical performance and work capacity by challenging different aspects of fitness, including strength, endurance, power, agility, speed, flexibility, coordination, and balance.

Mixed-mode training may not be the most effective method for building maximal strength or heaps of muscle, but it can be effective for those looking to lose fat while maintaining the muscle they have. If programmed effectively with the appropriate intensity, as with the programs found in this chapter, mixed-mode training forces you to focus on significant strength training and consistently challenge the muscle you have.

Using mixed-mode training to improve work capacity can also be an extremely time-efficient and effective way to prevent boredom for those who may not love the slower pace of traditional strength training. However, it's important to approach mixed-mode training with proper technique, gradually progress in intensity and complexity, and be smart with exercise selection.

Work Capacity

In the context of fitness, *work capacity* refers to the ability of an individual to perform a certain amount of physical work over a given period of time. It represents the overall capacity of the body to tolerate and sustain effort during various activities and is closely related to stamina.

Work capacity encompasses the combined elements of muscular strength, cardiovascular fitness, power, and endurance. It reflects how efficiently the body can generate and sustain energy, as well as how effectively it can tolerate and recover from physical exertion. Higher work capacity enables individuals to perform tasks with greater efficiency, endure longer periods of activity, and withstand physical demands without experiencing excessive fatigue.

Training for work capacity often involves exercises or workouts that challenge multiple muscle groups simultaneously, such as circuit training, or the complexes and combinations found in this chapter. These activities help to improve overall muscular endurance, strength, and some cardiovascular fitness through enhanced oxygen delivery to muscles and improved energy production.

Ultimately, increased work capacity enables individuals to perform physical tasks more effectively with reduced fatigue. It can also be advantageous in both athletic performance and daily activities requiring sustained effort.

Frequency

The ability to recover from training can become a limiting factor when it comes to implementing mixed-mode or work capacity–focused training too often. Overusing the same muscles and movements too frequently can lead to injury risk and overuse. With this in mind, we recommend using the advanced conditioning examples and programs found in this chapter no more than two to three times a week consistently. You will also find that some of the sequences included may serve as great additions to include in (rather than replace) more traditional strength work, such as adding a landmine complex from this chapter to the end of a hypertrophy or strength program in the following chapters.

Exercise Selection and Intensity

Not all exercises are created equal when programming effective conditioning sequences for improved work capacity and fat loss. The key is to prioritize compound movements that engage multiple muscle groups simultaneously. Exercises like squats, deadlifts, lunges, presses, and pulls are excellent choices because they require coordinated effort from various muscle groups.

These compound exercises not only stimulate a greater metabolic response than their isolation counterparts (think bicep curls and calf raises) but if done with challenging loads can aid in maintaining muscle mass and strength levels. The landmine can be a great tool for this style of training because of the ease of transition from one exercise to the next; however, pairing the right exercises together takes some strategy to best account for weight transitions between exercises. Circuits may allow for more time to change weights between movements, whereas complexes are meant to be done with no rest or weight transition between exercises.

ADVANCED CONDITIONING CIRCUITS

Circuit training is widespread, but to maximize the goals discussed here, the use of the right formula and appropriate pairing of landmine exercises is important for delivering big results. The circuits described here in tables 9.1, 9.2, and 9.3 are a great place to start, but because we want you to know how to build your own, you'll find that we have also included the movement category framework used so that you can adapt them and evolve as you see fit. Exercises not featured in this book have been denoted "N/A" and can be easily looked up for full context.

Here are a few overarching key points regarding these workouts that will help you get the most out of them and adapt them as needed over time:

Rest
- Ideally, rest is kept to 15 to 20 seconds between exercises.
- Once the entire circuit has been completed, then rest for 60 to 90 seconds; you can progress to the shorter end of that range over time.

Reps/Time
- These workouts can be performed for reps or time depending on your training level and preference.
- Using reps can be a great way to introduce these workouts because it may be easier to estimate the weights to use. However, over time, transitioning to time-based programming may increase the intensity of the circuit and for many exercisers can result in increased work intensity.

Sets

- Start by performing any of the following circuits for three rounds and progress up to four or five as desired.

Intensity

- Using a scale of 1 to 10, with 10 being near maximum effort, you should work to a 7 or 8 on the intensity scale with each exercise. This should allow for quality form throughout the set whether you are doing reps or time.
- It can be challenging to estimate weights if transitioning from traditional strength work. Keep in mind that you will do multiple rounds and will likely increase and fine-tune the weights after the first round of a circuit.
- Try and select exercises that use similar weights while maintaining challenge on the muscles or movements and, if necessary, make quick weight transitions during your rest period.

Substitute when necessary

- Great training programs are not about handcuffing you to exercises that aren't right for your body. If you find yourself in pain or uncomfortable with an exercise, don't force it.

Chapter 7 talks about the concept of individuality, and we had this in mind when we built out the programming options that follow. We have included movement patterns in the workout programs that match the exercises listed in earlier chapters in the book to give you programming options and the ability to adapt. Some moves may just not fit your body and how it moves. Simply choose another exercise option in that movement category that you can perform through the full range of motion without pain.

Table 9.1   Advanced Total Body Circuit A

Exercise	Page	Movement	Reps or time	Rest
(A1) Staggered single-arm press	44	Push	12 reps or 30 sec per side	15 sec
(A2) Landmine goblet squat	82	Squat	12 reps or 30 sec	15 sec
(A3) Staggered Meadows row	72	Pull	12 reps or 30 sec per side	15 sec
(A4) Rainbows	188	Core	12 reps/side or 30 sec total	60-90 sec

Table 9.2   Advanced Total Body Circuit B

Exercise	Page	Movement	Reps or time	Rest
(A1) Staggered single-arm row	68	Pull	12 reps or 30 sec per side	15 sec
(A2) Landmine thruster	144	Full body	12 reps or 30 sec total	15 sec
(A3) Landmine bear crawl	197	Core	30-60 sec	15 sec
(A4) Running/rowing/biking	N/A	Cardio	60-90 sec	60-90 sec

Table 9.3 Advanced Total Body Circuit C

Exercise	Page	Movement	Reps or time	Rest
(A1) Push press	166	Push	12 reps or 30 sec per side	15 sec
(A2) Bottom-loaded reverse lunge	110	Lunge	12 reps or 30 sec total	15 sec
(A3) Two-handed landmine row (prison row)	64	Pull	12 reps or 30 sec per side	15 sec
(A4) Landmine anchored dead-bug	176	Core	30-60 sec	60-90 sec

ADVANCED CONDITIONING COMPLEXES

In landmine training protocols, a *complex* refers to a series of exercise sets performed one after the other using a single piece of equipment. There are no breaks between movements, no changing weights, and you hold onto the equipment throughout. The number of reps can vary for each exercise, but generally, they're kept low. Completing a complex typically takes about 60 to 90 seconds. When selecting a weight for the complex, focus on challenging your weakest body parts to ensure balanced and effective training.

Here are a few overarching key points regarding the workouts in tables 9.4, 9.5, and 9.6 that will help you get the most out of them and adapt them as needed over time.

Rest

- There should be little to no rest between exercises—transition directly into the next exercise.
- Once the complex has been completed, rest for 60 to 90 seconds before attempting the complex again.
- Complexes can be extremely challenging. If you see performance drop drastically from set to set, then adjust your rest periods to allow for more recovery.

Reps or Time

- These workouts can be performed for reps or time depending on your training level and preference.
- Reps are not generally high for complexes. If programming for time, choose times that allow for 6 to 12 reps per exercise to still allow for challenging weights.

Sets

- These complexes can be done three to five times with rest in between.
- More advanced trainees may set a time of 15 to 20 minutes and challenge themselves to see how many quality rounds they can complete in the time allowed.

Intensity

- Using a scale of 1 to 10, with 10 being near maximum effort, you should work to a 7 or 8 on the intensity scale with each exercise. This should allow for quality form throughout the set whether you are doing reps or time.
- It can be challenging to estimate weights if transitioning from traditional strength work. Keep in mind that you will do multiple rounds will likely increase and fine-tune the weights after the first round of a circuit.
- Your goal should be to try and increase the loads you can handle over time rather than to complete the complexes faster.

Table 9.4   Advanced Total Body Complex A (Unilateral)

Exercise	Page	Movement	Reps or time	Rest
(A1) Single-arm press	42	Push	6-8 reps or 20 sec per side	N/A
(A2) Offset surfer squat	90	Squat	6-8 reps or 20 sec per side	N/A
(A3) Meadows row	70	Pull	6-8 reps or 20 sec per side	N/A
(A4) Bottom-loaded reverse lunge	110	Lunge	6-8 reps or 20 sec per side	60-90 sec

Complete all reps on one side of the body for each move simultaneously before moving to the opposite side.

Table 9.5   Advanced Total Body Complex B

Exercise	Page	Movement	Reps or time	Rest
(A1) Landmine thruster	144	Full body	10 reps or 30 sec	NA
(A2) Staggered single-arm press	44	Push	10 reps or 30 sec/side	NA
(A3) Single-leg RDL	132	Hinge	10 reps or 30 sec/side	NA
(A4) Meadows row	70	Pull	10 reps or 30 sec/side	NA

Table 9.6   Advanced Total Body Complex C

Exercise	Page	Movement	Reps or time	Rest
(A1) Angled landmine reverse lunge	112	Lunge	6 reps	NA
(A2) Staggered RDL	128	Hinge	6 reps	NA
(A3) Single-arm press	42	Push	6 reps	NA
(A4) Staggered row	N/A	Pull	6 reps	60-90 sec

Complete all reps on one side of the body for each move simultaneously before moving to the opposite side.

ADVANCED CONDITIONING WITH TRAINING SPLITS (THREE TIMES PER WEEK)

The circuits and complexes presented in the previous section can serve as time-efficient and brutally challenging stand-alone workouts, but they may better serve as an addition to a complete training program that allows for consistent hypertrophy and strength work. This can be a great way to maintain and even continue to gain in these areas while building work capacity with circuits and complexes. The programming in tables 9.7, 9.8, and 9.9 serves as an example framework for how these would fit together within a complete training program with both landmine and other traditional exercises.

Table 9.7   Advanced Conditioning Workout A (Upper Body Push Focus)

Exercise	Page	Movement	Week 1	Week 2	Week 3	Week 4
(A) Kneeling land-mine press	48	Push	3 × 8	4 × 6-8	4 × 6-8	5 × 6
(B1) Single-arm floor press	60	Push	3 × 12/ side	3× 10-12/ side	3 × 10-12/ side	3 × 8-10/ side
(B2) Push-ups	N/A	Push	3 × 15	3 × 15	3× max	3× max
(C) Circuit or complex of choice for three to five rounds.						

Table 9.8   Advanced Conditioning Workout B (Lower Body Focus)

Exercise	Page	Movement	Week 1	Week 2	Week 3	Week 4
(A) Landmine goblet squat	82	Squat	3 × 8	4 × 6-8	4 × 6-8	5 × 6
(B1) Angled Zercher reverse lunge	113	Lunge	3 × 12/ side	3 × 10-12/ side	3 × 10-12/ side	3 × 8-10/ side
(B2) Staggered calf raise	140	Accessory	3 × 15/ side	3 × 15/ side	3 × 15/ side	3 × 15/ side
(C) Circuit or complex of choice for three to five rounds.						

Table 9.9   Advanced Conditioning Workout C (Upper Body Pull Focus)

Exercise	Page	Movement	Week 1	Week 2	Week 3	Week 4
(A) T-bar row	66	Pull	3 × 8	4 × 6-8	4 × 6-8	5 × 6
(B1) Staggered Meadows row	72	Pull	3 × 12/ side	3 × 10-12/ side	3 × 10-12/ side	3 × 8-10/ side
(B2) Concentration curl	78	Accessory	3 × 12/ side	3 × 12/ side	3 × 12/ side	3 × 12/ side
(C) Circuit or complex of choice for three to five rounds.						

Advanced conditioning with the landmine builds on the solid foundation established in the previous chapter, so make sure not to skip steps and jump in on these workouts without establishing a solid base. These workouts challenge multiple fitness components simultaneously, making them ideal for those who have already mastered the basics.

As you progress through these advanced conditioning programs, remember the importance of proper technique, gradual progression, and intelligent exercise selection. The following chapters will continue to provide you with targeted training plans geared toward your goals of building muscle, strength, and athleticism.

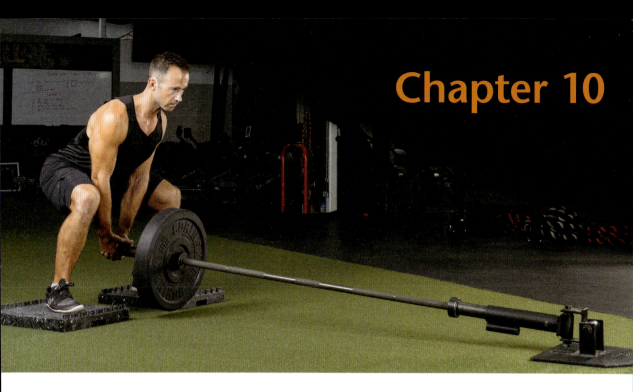

Chapter 10

HYPERTROPHY TRAINING

Want to look good naked? You're in the right place, but the advantages of building muscle are more than just skin-deep. Beyond boosting your appearance, muscular development, also known as hypertrophy, offers a range of benefits, including increased strength, improved metabolism, increased bone density, and even a longer lifespan.

This chapter introduces a straightforward approach to building muscle that is centered on the effective use of the landmine as a primary workout tool. Whether you're new to lifting or a seasoned bodybuilder, the workouts in this chapter can level up your training.

MUSCLE-BUILDING PRINCIPLES

Many training methods can effectively build muscle, but they all stem from a core set of proven principles. Follow these principles and you should continue to see lasting results, regardless of the training tool.

Rep Ranges and the Role of Failure

There's no one-size-fits-all rep range for effectively building muscle. Research shows that both low-rep and higher-rep ranges can be used as long as the sets are performed to failure (Schoenfeld 2017). This means that sets of 12 to 20 reps can be just as effective as sets of 1 to 5 reps as long as they are performed at or close to mechanical failure (i.e., 1 rep in the tank). What's important, regardless of the rep range, is that the focus is on mechanical tension.

Although all rep ranges may be fair game for hypertrophy training, the extremes may not be practical for all exercisers. Learning to truly train to failure while not sacrificing technique is a skill—one that takes time to get right. If you train too heavy with low rep ranges, the quality of your reps can be hard to maintain. Alternatively, hitting failure with extremely high rep sets takes a lot of trial and error, can be tough on joints, and, when done correctly, can be so brutal it's not enjoyable.

This is why you will find reps between 6 and 15 in the example programs that follow. Training close to failure in this range tends to be most practical for the widest range of exercisers and still leaves significant room for variation.

Exercise Tempo

There is a time for moving fast and being explosive, but if the focus is on mechanical tension to build muscle, then the key is to slow it down and minimize momentum. The concentric (lifting) portion of every rep should be performed at a normal tempo (one to two seconds), while the lowering phase of the exercise should be even slower. Evidence supports the benefit of slowing down the eccentric (lowering) phase to a rate of three to four seconds to maximize mechanical tension and drive muscle growth (Pereria et al. 2016). Armed with this information, you should aim to perform every rep in a controlled manner with a two- to three-second lowering and one-second lifting tempo.

Training Frequency and Sets

The easiest way to look at training frequency has to do with the realistic number of days each week you can and want to strength train. For those with less training experience or time, two- to three-day-a-week routines are best suited for a full body approach. For those with more training experience and higher-level physique goals, an upper body, lower body training split four days a week may be a better fit. We have included examples for both.

What seems to matter most for increasing muscle size is that you train 12 to 20 total sets per muscle each week. This can be split several ways, but it should help provide a guide as to whether you are training muscles enough or too much throughout the week.

FUNCTIONAL BODYBUILDING

Functional bodybuilding is a newly popular term in the industry to describe a training approach that combines traditional bodybuilding exercises with more functional movements. Without diving back into the functional training debate mentioned in chapter 2, the term might be great as a way to think about how landmine exercises fit into a muscle-building program.

The functional bodybuilding concept effectively highlights the relevance of the stability continuum introduced in chapter 1. Training along various points on this continuum can offer significant long-term benefits, but too much instability can be detrimental to maintaining the mechanical tension necessary to drive muscle growth.

If your goal is to build muscle, then your takeaway is to make sure you are choosing landmine exercises, loads, and reps that allow you to maintain controlled tension on the specific muscles you are targeting. Not all exercises are equal here because of the impact of instability on muscular tension, especially if you haven't already established a solid base of training with the landmine.

UNLEASH MUSCLE GROWTH WITH THE LANDMINE

Building legitimate muscle mass takes time, but follow either of the example programs included in this chapter and you will be well on your way to noticeable gains in muscle size. The first routine is meant to be done two to three times a week and takes a full body approach with the landmine as your primary training tool. The second program is built around an upper and lower body split geared toward training four times a week and incorporates other common gym equipment as well.

Here are a few overarching key points regarding these workouts that will help you get the most out of them and adapt them as needed over time.

Rest

- In general, resting one to two minutes between sets is ideal for building muscle because the final sets will be performed closer to failure.
- For the programs included here, we recommend resting for at least 90 seconds after each complete set before repeating the next.

Reps

- The priority here is controlled and intentional execution of each rep with perfect technique.
- We will train at the lower and higher ends of the hypertrophy rep ranges; the key is to maintain tempo and adjust loads to best fit the rep range for each exercise. This may take you a few sets, or even weeks, to figure out.

Intensity

- Effectively building muscle means learning what it's like to safely train to failure. The first set of each exercise can be a "building" set. By the time you reach the last one to two sets, you should have no more than one more rep in the tank when complete.
- Using a scale of 0 to 10, with 10 representing total failure, your goal should be to work up to 8 to 10 on your final sets in each of the following workouts.

Substitute when necessary

- Great training programs are not about handcuffing you to exercises that aren't right for your body. If you find yourself in pain or uncomfortable with an exercise, don't force it.
- Chapter 7 talks about the concept of individuality, and we had this in mind when we built out the programming options that follow. We have included movement patterns in the workout programs that match the exercises listed in earlier chapters in the book to give you programming options and the ability to adapt. Some moves may just not fit your body and how it moves. Simply choose another exercise option in that movement category that you can perform through the full range of motion without pain.

FULL BODY LANDMINE-ONLY PROGRAM

This first training program in tables 10.1, 10.2, and 10.3 serves as a complete total body hypertrophy template that could be repeated and progressed with loads for at least two to three months. The programs in this chapter are meant to be flexible with the inclusion of the movement categories so you can choose the right version of each pattern for you, but we do recommend sticking to the same primary pattern for no fewer than eight weeks before changing it. This is necessary to get good enough at the exercises to effectively train close to failure within the reps prescribed. Most of these programs are set up in superset-style for workout efficiency but they could also be done as single-exercise sets. Exercises that are not featured in this book will be denoted with "N/A" and may be easily looked up for more context.

Table 10.1   Hypertrophy Total Body A (Hinging + Pressing Dominant)

Exercise	Page	Movement	Week 1	Week 2	Week 3	Week 4
(A1) Landmine sumo deadlift	136	Hinge	3 × 6-8	4 × 6-8	5 × 6	5 ×6
(A2) Half-kneeling single-arm press	50	Push	3 × 6-8	4 × 6-8	5 × 6	5 ×6
(B1) Staggered RDL	128	Hinge	3 × 10-12/ side	3 × 10-12/ side	3 × 10/ side	4 × 10/ side
(B2) Standing two-arm landmine press	38	Push	3 × 10-12	3 × 10-12	3 × 10-12	4 × 10
(C1) Single-arm floor press	60	Push	3 × 15	3 × 15	3 × 15	3 × 15
(C2) Standing calf raise	138	Accessory	3 × 15	3 × 15	3 × 15	3 × 15
(C3) Landmine roll-out	192	Core	3 × 10-12	3 × 10-12	3 × 10-12	3 × 10-12

Table 10.2   Hypertrophy Total Body B (Lunging + Pulling Dominant)

Exercise	Page	Movement	Week 1	Week 2	Week 3	Week 4
(A1) Elevated reverse lunge	106	Lunge	3 × 6-8/ side	4 × 6-8/ side	5 × 6/ side	5 × 6/ side
(A2) Staggered Meadows row	72	Pull	3 × 6-8/ side	4 × 6-8/ side	5 × 6/ side	5 × 6/ side
(B1) Angled Zercher reverse lunge	113	Lunge	3 × 10-12/ side	3 × 10-12/ side	3 × 10/ side	4 × 10/ side
(B2) T-bar row (with towel)	66	Pull	3 × 10-12	3 × 10-12	3 × 10-12	4 × 10
(C1) Sissy squat	94	Squat	3 × 15	3 × 15	3 × 15	3 × 15
(C2) Concentration curl	78	Accessory	3 × 15	3 × 15	3 × 15	3 × 15
(C3) Rainbows	188	Core	3 × 10/ side	3 × 10/ side	3 × 10/ side	3 × 10/ side

Table 10.3 Hypertrophy Total Body C (Squatting + Push/pull)

Exercise	Page	Movement	Week 1	Week 2	Week 3	Week 4
(A1) Landmine goblet squat	82	Squat	3 × 6-8	4 × 6-8	5 × 6	5 × 6
(B1) Staggered single-arm press	44	Push	3 × 10/side	3 × 8/side	4 × 8/side	4 × 6/side
(B2) Two-handed landmine row (prison row)	64	Pull	3 × 10/side	3 × 8/side	4 × 8/side	4 × 6/side
(C1) Offset squat	86	Squat	3 × 10/side	3 × 10/side	3 × 10/side	3 × 10/side
(C2) Kneeling landmine press	48	Push	3 × 10-12	3 × 10-12	3 × 10-12	3 × 10-12
(D1) Hack squat	88	Squat	3 × 15	3 × 15	3 × 15	3 × 15
(D2) Mixed-grip curl	79	Accessory	3 × 12/side	3 × 12/side	3 × 12/side	3 × 12/side

LANDMINE-INTEGRATED PROGRAMS

The program example that follows in tables 10.4, 10.5, 10.6, and 10.7 is best suited for exercisers who have performed hypertrophy training programs before and require more focused body part–specific volume for increased muscle growth. The four-day split may also be better suited for those who enjoy more frequent strength training each week. The landmine-only programs included in this book are very effective, but they may be limited when it comes to the single-joint isolation work that is more prevalent in bodybuilding.

The following program has also been built around the movement categories already mentioned to allow for flexibility and uses commonly found gym equipment (cables, dumbbells, barbells, and the landmine). The four workouts are designed so that workouts A and B could be performed on consecutive days, followed by a day of rest from strength training. Then, workouts C and D could be performed again on the following two consecutive days, with one to two days of rest before cycling back to workout A.

Table 10.4   Hypertrophy Workout A (Lower Body 1)

Exercise	Page	Movement	Week 1	Week 2	Week 3	Week 4
(A1) RFE split squat	118	Lunge	3 × 6-8/ side	4 × 6-8/ side	5 × 6/ side	5 × 6/ side
(B1) Landmine goblet squat	82	Squat	3 × 10-12	3 × 10	4 × 8	4 × 8
(B2) Hamstring curl machine *or* stability ball	N/A	Accessory Hinge	3 × 12	3 × 12	4 × 10	4 × 10
(C1) Adductor RDL	126	Hinge	3 × 10-12	3 × 10-12	3 × 10-12	3 × 10-12
(C2) Leg extension	N/A	Accessory Push	3 × 15	3 × 15	3 × 15	3 × 15
(D1) Dumbbell walking lunges	N/A	Lunge	3 × 15/ side	3 × 15/ side	3 × 12/ side	3 × 12/ side
(D2) Staggered calf raise	140	Accessory	3 × 15/ side	3 × 15/ side	3 × 15/ side	3 × 15/ side

Table 10.5   Hypertrophy Workout B (Upper Body 1)

Exercise	Page	Movement	Week 1	Week 2	Week 3	Week 4
(A1) Staggered Meadows row	72	Pull	3 × 6-8/ side	4 × 6-8/ side	5 × 6/ side	5 × 6/ side
(B1) Standing two-arm landmine press	38	Push	3 × 8-10	3 × 8	4 × 8	4 × 8
(B2) Lat pull-down	N/A	Pull	3 × 12	3 × 12	4 × 10	4 × 10
(C1) Dumbbell chest press	N/A	Push	3 × 10-12	3 × 10-12	3 × 10-12	3 × 10-12
(C2) T-bar row	66	Pull	3 × 15	3 × 15	3 × 15	3 × 15
(D1) Dumbbell curl	N/A	Accessory	3 × 12-15	3 × 12-15	3 × 12-15	3 × 12-15
(D2) Cable triceps	N/A	Accessory	3 × 12-15	3 × 12-15	3 × 12-15	3 × 12-15

Table 10.6   Hypertrophy Workout C (Lower Body 2)

Exercise	Page	Movement	Week 1	Week 2	Week 3	Week 4
(A1) Staggered RDL	128	Hinge	3 × 6-8/ side	4 × 6-8/ side	5 × 6/ side	5 × 6/ side
(B1) Angled Zercher reverse lunge	113	Lunge	3 × 10-12/ side	3 × 10-12/ side	4 × 8/ side	4 × 8/ side
(B2) Standing calf raise	138	Accessory	3 × 12-15	3 × 12-15	4 × 12	4 × 12
(C1) Elevated reverse lunge	106	Lunge	3 × 12/ side	3 × 12/ side	3 × 12/ side	3 × 12/ side
(C2) Cable kickback	N/A	Accessory Hinge	3 × 15/ side	3 × 15/ side	3 × 15/ side	3 × 15/ side
(D1) Heels-elevated cyclist squat	N/A	Squat	3 × 15	3 × 15	3 × 15	3 × 15
(D2) Landmine anchored reverse crunch	178	Core	3 × 12-15	3 × 12-15	3 × 12-15	3 × 12-15

Table 10.7   Hypertrophy Workout D (Upper Body 2)

Exercise	Page	Movement	Week 1	Week 2	Week 3	Week 4
(A1) Staggered single-arm press	44	Push	3 × 6-8/ side	4 × 6-8/ side	5 × 6/ side	5 × 6/ side
(B1) Meadows row	70	Pull	3 × 8-10/ side	3 × 8/side	4 × 8/ side	4 × 8/ side
(B2) Standing shoulder-to-shoulder press	40	Push	3 × 10/ side	3 × 12/ side	4 × 10/ side	4 × 10/ side
(C1) Pull-ups	N/A	Pull	3 × 10-12	3 × 10-12	3 × 10-12	3 × 10-12
(C2) Cable chest fly	N/A	Push	3 × 15	3 × 15	3 × 15	3 × 15
(D1) Mixed-grip curl	79	Accessory	3 × 12-15/ side	3 × 12-15/ side	3 × 12-15/ side	3 × 12-15/ side
(D2) Dumbbell skull-crushers	N/A	Accessory	3 × 12-15	3 × 12-15	3 × 12-15	3 × 12-15

Hypertrophy training with the landmine offers a comprehensive and effective approach to building muscle and achieving a well-rounded physique. By adhering to principles such as proper rep ranges, controlled tempo, and appropriate training frequency, you can maximize muscle growth and even have some spillover into strength.

The programs in this chapter are designed to suit both beginners and experienced lifters, ensuring that everyone can benefit from the landmine's versatility. As you progress through these workouts, stay focused on maintaining form and pushing toward controlled failure to achieve the best results.

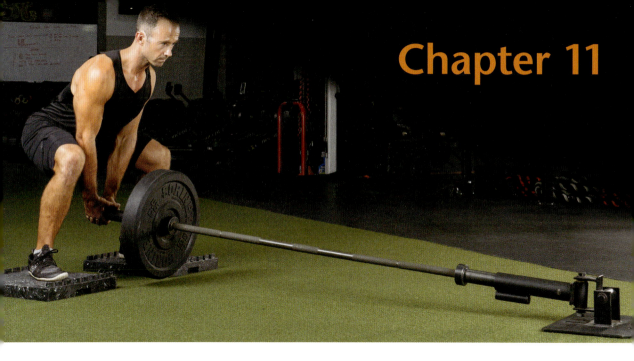

Chapter 11

STRENGTH DEVELOPMENT

While the training programs discussed in previous chapters lay the groundwork for physical prowess, the development of strength throughout your training journey is crucial. Building greater strength goes beyond aesthetics and athletic performance, offering a myriad of benefits, from enhanced functional capacity to longevity. This chapter lays out a pragmatic approach to building strength, spotlighting the landmine as a primary tool.

The term *maximal strength* refers to the capacity to exert as much force as possible. It is distinct from power, focusing on the sustained application of force rather than its rapid generation. While power training, described in chapter 12, often involves high-velocity movements, maximal strength serves as an important precursor.

A fair amount of confusion often surrounds how to differentiate hypertrophy, strength, and power. It's not as though a switch goes off or on when transitioning from building muscle to strength or strength to power. It would be easier if this were the case, but there will likely be a fair amount of crossover as you train long term and make your way through programs like those in this book. Think about the various training phases and goals like a

VIP rope, as shown in figure 11.1. If you pull upward on any part of the rope, it's not only going to raise the rope where your hand is but also the areas around it.

The key is to realize that it's about a shift in the primary intention. Building muscle means focusing on mechanical overload and metabolic stress. The resulting larger muscles increase the potential for strength, but then that potential has to be realized and maximized. Increasing strength means using heavier

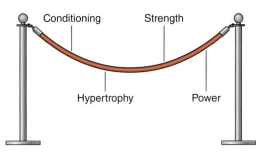

Figure 11.1   This rope is meant to visualize how your primary training focus will still likely have crossover into other improvements. Pull up on any section of the rope and it's going to also elevate the qualities around it.

loads that challenge the nervous system's ability to coordinate and recruit more muscle fibers all at the same time, resulting in improvements in the ability to generate force.

STRENGTH AS A SKILL

It's widely accepted that most true strength adaptations happen when working with weights 80 to 100 percent of one rep max, but learning to lift heavier loads safely and effectively also takes time. It should be seen as a skill that is best built upon a solid foundation of technique, stability, and familiarity with the exercises being performed. Regardless of your training experience, landmine training is unique. As such, there is tremendous value in working through some of the previous programs to ensure that you have spent adequate time on the movements and have developed the skills necessary to lift heavy. Heavier loads can increase risk and strain on the body, so we want technique and execution to be perfect.

This skill element is also one of the reasons you will find most of the strength work in this chapter in the 80 to 90 percent range, rather than at or near true one rep max levels. Absolute one rep maximal strength has value, but chances are you didn't pick up this landmine training book because you want to compete in powerlifting. You likely want to move better, avoid injury, and increase your ability to do the things you enjoy in life and at the gym. None of that requires training for one rep maxes. The risk isn't likely worth the reward, so rather than reach true failure you will find rep ranges and programming that allow for building adequate strength and maximal fiber recruitment while maintaining a focus on quality movement and safety, primarily in the three to six rep range.

IMPORTANCE OF BUILDING STRENGTH

Outside of athletics and the powerlifting world, true strength is often undervalued in the broader fitness landscape. Its significance extends beyond competitive sports, directly influencing daily activities and longevity. Developing higher levels of relative strength aids in injury prevention, enhances bone density, and fortifies connective tissues.

Many people may shy away from training in strength-building zones because they associate it only with specific lifts such as barbell squatting, bench pressing, and deadlifting, and these movements may not feel great on the body. The landmine offers a variety of unique alternative movements and positions that may be better suited for those looking to increase strength without pain and those who may be working around long-standing limitations.

BUILDING A STRENGTH PROGRAM WITH THE LANDMINE

Frequency recommendations can vary widely based on training levels and preferences, but to stick with the compound lift and movement category approach seen in the book so far, we have included both three- and four-times-per-week sample programs. Here are a few overarching key points regarding these workouts that will help you get the most out of them and adapt them as needed over time:

Rest

- Rest times may vary throughout a training session based on whether you are doing the initial main strength lifts or accessory work, but rest periods should be no less than two to three minutes between main strength sets to maximize recovery.
- Note your performance from set to set and increase the rest times if performance or strength drop significantly.

Reps/Time

- The priority here is controlled and intentional execution of each rep with perfect technique.
- At least one to two primary strength lifts will be performed in the three to six rep range, but the number of reps for accessory supporting lifts will vary.

Intensity

- It's unlikely that you will know one rep maxes to program from, but you should be able to gauge relative three rep maxes for some of the main lifts to help with load selection.

- If you think of your intensity on a scale from 0 to 10, with 10 representing total failure, then your goal should be to work up to 8 to 9 on the majority of working sets.
- You can build significant strength without hitting failure, so be patient and maintain high-quality technique.

Substitute when necessary

- Great training programs are not about handcuffing you to exercises that aren't right for your body. If you find yourself in pain or uncomfortable with an exercise, don't force it.
- We have included movement patterns in the workouts that match the exercises listed previously in the book to give you programming options and the ability to adapt. Simply choose another regression or progression that you can perform through the full range of motion without pain.

FULL BODY LANDMINE-ONLY PROGRAM

This first training program in tables 11.1, 11.2, and 11.3 serves as a complete three-day-per-week total body strength template that could be repeated and progressed with loads for at least two to three months. This would mean cycling back to week one variables after completing week four. These programs are meant to be flexible with the inclusion of the movement categories so you can choose the right version of each pattern for you, but we do recommend sticking to the same primary patterns for no less than eight weeks before changing them. This is necessary to get good enough at the exercises to effectively load them and create the desired neurological adaptations. These programs include more straight sets in the beginning and then finish with supersets.

Table 11.1   Strength Total Body A (Hinging + Pressing Dominant)

Exercise	Page	Movement	Week 1	Week 2	Week 3	Week 4
(A1) Landmine sumo deadlift	136	Hinge	4 × 5	5 × 5	6 × 4	3 × 8
(B1) Kneeling landmine press	48	Push	4 × 5	5 × 5	6 × 4	3 × 8
(C1) Staggered RDL	128	Hinge	3 × 8/ side	3 × 8/ side	3 × 8/ side	3 × 12-15/ side
(C2) Single-arm press	42	Push	3 × 8/ side	3 × 8/ side	3 × 8/ side	3 × 12-15/ side
(D1) Single-arm floor press	60	Push	3 × 12/ side	3 × 12/ side	3 × 12/ side	3 × 15/ side
(D2) Rainbows	188	Core	3 × 10	3 × 10	3 × 10	3 × 10

Table 11.2   Strength Total Body B (Lunging + Pulling Dominant)

Exercise	Page	Movement	Week 1	Week 2	Week 3	Week 4
(A1) Elevated reverse lunge	106	Lunge	4 × 6/ side	5 × 5/ side	6 × 4/ side	3 × 8/ side
(B1) Staggered Meadows row (supported)	72	Pull	4 × 6/ side	5 × 5/ side	6 × 4/ side	3 × 8/ side
(C1) Static lateral lunge	98	Lunge	3 × 8-10/ side	3 × 8-10/ side	3 × 8-10/ side	3 × 12/ side
(C2) T-bar row (with towel)	66	Pull	3 × 8-10	3 × 8-10	3 × 8-10	3 × 15
(D1) Sissy squat	94	Squat	3 × 12	3 × 12	3 × 12	3 × 15
(C2) Lateral raise	77	Accessory	3 × 12-15/ side	3 × 12-15	3 × 12-15	3 × 12-15

Table 11.3   Strength Total Body C (Squatting + Push/pull)

Exercise	Page	Movement	Week 1	Week 2	Week 3	Week 4
(A1) Landmine goblet squat	82	Squat	4 × 6	5 × 5	6 × 4	3 × 8
(B1) Staggered single-arm press	44	Push	4 × 6/side	5 × 5/ side	6 × 4/ side	3 × 8/ side
(C1) Staggered single-arm row	68	Pull	3 × 8/side	3 × 8/ side	3 × 8/ side	3 × 12/ side
(C2) Offset surfer squat	90	Squat	3 × 8/side	3 × 8/ side	3 × 8/ side	3 × 12/ side
(D1) Kneeling push press	150	Full body	3 × 12	3 × 12	3 × 12	3 × 15
(D2) Hack squat	88	Squat	3 × 12	3 × 12	3 × 12	3 × 15
(D3) Landmine anchored reverse crunch	178	Core	3 × 12	3 × 12	3 × 12	3 × 12

LANDMINE-INTEGRATED PROGRAMS

The program example that follows in tables 11.4, 11.5, 11.6, and 11.7 is best suited to trainees who have trained extensively in the past and who may require more recovery time between training repeat movements and muscles. The four-day split may also be better suited for those who enjoy more frequent strength training each week. The landmine-only programs included in this book are brutally effective, but may be limited by things like position and grip when it comes to training heavy.

The program that follows has also been built around the movement categories to allow for flexibility and uses commonly found gym equipment: cables, dumbbells, barbells, and the landmine. The four workouts are designed so that workouts A and B could be performed on consecutive days, followed by a day of rest from strength training. Then, workouts C and D could be performed again on the following two consecutive days, with one to two days of rest before cycling back to workout A. If looking to stay consistent with this program for 8 to 12 weeks, then repeat by cycling back to week one variables after completing week four.

Table 11.4   Strength Workout A (Lower Body 1)

Exercise	Page	Movement	Week 1	Week 2	Week 3	Week 4
(A1) RFE split squat	118	Lunge	4 × 6/side	5 × 5/side	6 × 4/side	3 × 8/side
(B1) Landmine goblet squat	82	Squat	4 × 8	4 × 6	5 × 5	3 × 8
(C1) Staggered RDL	128	Hinge	3 × 8-10/side	3 × 8-10/side	3 × 8-10/side	3 × 8-10/side
(C2) Leg extension	N/A	Accessory Push	3 × 10	3 × 10	3 × 10	3 × 10
(D1) Dumbbell lateral lunge	N/A	Lunge	3 × 12/side	3 × 12/side	3 × 12/side	3 × 12/side
(D2) Rainbows	188	Core	3 × 10/side	3 × 10/side	3 × 10/side	3 × 10/side

Table 11.5   Strength Workout B (Upper Body 1)

Exercise	Page	Movement	Week 1	Week 2	Week 3	Week 4
(A1) Staggered Meadows row	72	Pull	4 × 6/side	5 × 5/side	6 × 4/side	3 × 8/side
(B1) Dumbbell bench press	N/A	Push	4 × 5	5 × 5	6 × 4	3 × 8
(C1) Lat pulldown	N/A	Pull	3 × 8	3 × 8	3 × 8-10	3 × 8-10
(C2) Standing two-arm landmine press	38	Push	3 × 8	3 × 8	3 × 8-10	3 × 8-10
(D1) T-bar row (with towel)	66	Pull	3 × 12	3 × 12	3 × 12	3 × 15
(D2) Cable triceps	N/A	Accessory	3 × 12-15	3 × 12-15	3 × 12-15	3 × 12-15

Table 11.6 Strength Workout C (Lower Body 2)

Exercise	Page	Movement	Week 1	Week 2	Week 3	Week 4
(A1) Barbell hip thrust	N/A	Hinge	4 × 6	5 × 5	6 × 3-4	3 × 8
(B1) Angled Zercher reverse lunge	113	Lunge	4 × 8/side	4 × 6/side	5 × 5/side	3 × 8/side
(C1) Heels-elevated squat	84	Squat	3 × 10	3 × 10	3 × 10	3 × 10
C2) Hamstring curls or glute–ham developer	N/A	Accessory Hinge	3 × 10	3 × 10	3 × 10	3 × 10
(D1) Dumbbell walking lunges	N/A	Lunge	3 × 12/side	3 × 12/side	3 × 12/side	3 × 12/side
(D2) Landmine anchored leg lift	180	Core	3 × 10	3 × 10	3 × 10	3 × 10

Table 11.7 Strength Workout D (Upper Body 2)

Exercise	Page	Movement	Week 1	Week 2	Week 3	Week 4
(A1) Staggered single-arm press	44	Push	4 × 6/side	5 × 5/side	6 × 4/side	3 × 8/side
(B1) Single-arm dumbbell row	N/A	Pull	4 × 6/side	5 × 5/side	6 × 5/side	3 × 8/side
(C1) Barbell or dumbbell incline bench press	N/A	Push	3 × 8	3 × 8	3 × 8-10	3 × 8-10
(C2) Pull-ups (assisted or weighted)	N/A	Pull	3 × 8	3 × 8	3 × 8-10	3 × 8-10
(D1) Lateral raise	77	Pull Accessory	3 × 12/side	3 × 12	3 × 12	3 × 15
(D2) Rainbows	188	Core	3 × 12/side	3 × 12/side	3 × 12/side	3 × 12/side

Training for and developing maximal strength with the landmine is a skill that takes time. By focusing on proper technique, appropriate load management, and the right exercise selection, you can safely and efficiently build significant strength.

The programs in this chapter are designed to cater to both novice and experienced lifters, ensuring progressive overload while also offering a lot of training variety.

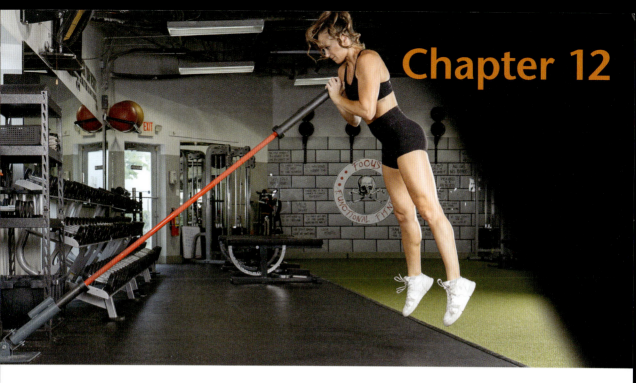

POWER TRAINING

The development of muscular power is important not just for athletes, but for everyone. Although many of these capabilities are task-dependent, training with speed and explosiveness has major benefits for the muscular and neurological systems. Previous chapters have built upon the skill and coordination components of training with the landmine, so in this chapter we can focus on generating force quickly.

Power training might be the most undervalued aspect of resistance training today. Although the benefits of strength training are becoming more well-known, few are preaching the benefits of performing strength-based movements with speed.

Explosive movements are required in both calculated and reactive scenarios—meaning when we are both planning to do something athletic as well as reacting to the world around us. This could be the fastball from the mound of a softball athlete or catching yourself from falling off of a curb—power is power. Regardless of the varying demands among demographic groups, a strong foundation of research shows the benefits of power training for muscular capacity and bone and connective tissue health (Hong and Kim 2018; Stone 1988).

The landmine is unique because training power can be introduced with ease and a customized approach due to its ability to pivot and be trained in locomotive situations. Researchers suggest that people implement a variety of training types to see the benefits of resistance training as they age (Torre and Temprado 2022).

WHAT IS POWER?

Strength training has long been promoted for its application to everyday tasks. Although strength training falls under the same umbrella of resistance training as power training, it is imperative to stress the importance of power for movement and quality of life. Muscular power is the generation of a high magnitude of force in a short period of time. This is what we would associate with more athletic movements in our day-to-day lives. Although most people aren't engaged in competitive athletics after the age of 40, that doesn't mean that those movement characteristics should be neglected.

Power generation is neuromuscular coordination. Because the body has varying demands on it on a daily basis, it's beneficial to learn how to handle both the production and absorption of power throughout the body. Power production is most commonly seen in reactive scenarios. However, to protect our joints, the ability to absorb force is just as important for long-term health.

WHY POWER MATTERS

One of the most common misconceptions is the notion that power capabilities are unique to sports performance settings. Unfortunately, this thought process may be the reason we see so many individuals who suffer from chronic pain and avoidable issues simply because they weren't aware of its importance.

Power is critical to the body's ability to react. Our environment has many constantly changing variables that we must adapt to. In this context, power training isn't just throwing a javelin or performing a kettlebell swing. For a first-time parent of a 9-month-old, power is what allows them to reach out at a moment's notice to catch their child from falling over. For the commuter, power can be the difference between catching the train to work or waiting for the next one. For the older adult, power can be the ability to drive their leg forward to catch themselves and prevent a fall.

As we come to understand power, specifically in regard to landmine training, it's important to understand that power varies from individual to individual. The power a 20-year-old athlete can generate will not be the same as that generated by a sedentary 72-year-old.

Landmine training has proven to be a beneficial modality in bridging the gap for individuals looking to enter into training protocols exploring power development and absorption. As expected, the unique stimulus of power training creates specific adaptations within the body.

POWER STARTS WITH STRENGTH

As previously mentioned, strength training is the foundation of power training, particularly for weight room–based activities. Generating high force in exercises with multiplied velocity can increase the risks associated with weight training if form and preparedness aren't taken into consideration. For this reason, it is recommended to begin training with a foundation of strength training before progressing to power-based movements. This approach allows for the achievement of the physiological, neuromuscular, and proprioceptive requirements needed to accommodate the introduction of velocity.

The programs provided in this chapter are a great way to generate power in your movements. As mentioned earlier, we recommend that you engage in a strength training routine and have quality movement patterning before progressing to a power-based program.

Due to the specific demands on the landmine, some of the areas that may need the most attention before progressing to power-based movements are:

- *Grip strength.* The width of the landmine is wider than the standard grip width seen with barbells, dumbbells, and kettlebells. Grabbing the end sleeve increases stress on the hand and wrist muscles.

- *Lateral instability.* Because the landmine can shift side to side when performing primarily linear movements, single-leg and core stability should be developed before introducing power movements.

- *Pattern angle.* The unique angle of the landmine can be a challenging new addition to an exerciser's skillset. This becomes increasingly important when transitioning to power movements.

Strength training has been shown to build the foundation for our physiological capacity. The logical progression from strength training is introducing power and building the characteristics to support it from both a muscular and neurological approach. As mentioned earlier, this becomes a focus of both the production and absorption of such power. Muscular strength across the body and localized to specific joints lays the foundation for a more resilient body.

BUILDING A POWER PROGRAM WITH THE LANDMINE

Power programming can typically be viewed as a less frequent mode of training than strength training. Whereas strength training is recommended anywhere from three to six times per week, power training is recommended two to three days per week. This difference in prescription is based on the neuromuscular demands of power training. Load management is an important component of any program. As previously mentioned, grip strength can be the most vulnerable area for technique error. When programming movements, it is important to consider grip demand across the spectrum of exercises selected.

One important benefit of the landmine is the ease of dumping the weight in the instance of a failed lift. This may be a factor that falls under the radar for many lifts, but it's always important to take into consideration the safety protocol.

Programming schemes have been broken down for you in previous chapters to apply in these areas. Because force generation is specific between regions of the body, programming should have an even distribution of power development from upper and lower body perspectives, as long as there are no contraindications.

A fundamental way to look at the power training methods available for programming is by breaking them down into linear power training and rotational power training.

LINEAR POWER TRAINING

Moving weight through a straight path via level changes is a great way to generate high levels of force production, muscular stress, and physiological demand during a workout. Generating enough energy to compete against gravity is one of the most fundamental methods of power training. More traditional methods such as Olympic lifts can be varied in iterations of their patterns with the landmine, as discussed in earlier chapters.

Linear methods of power production are recommended for individuals who do not have specific contraindications to resistance training activities. Due to the variable movement profile of the landmine, the modality is a strong complement to both vertical and horizontal movements. This can be helpful for those looking to build explosive components as part of their vertical profile (i.e., vertical jump performance), as well as integrating pieces of frontal plane work (i.e., lateral bounding). Tables 12.1 through 12.4 provide various linear power training workouts.

Table 12.1   Full Body Power Workout 1

Exercise	Page	Sets	Reps	Load
Single-arm clean (to press)	154	3-5	3-5	30-70% 1RM
Landmine sumo deadlift	136	3	8-12	70-80% 1RM
Half-kneeling single-arm press	50	3	8-12/side	70-80% 1RM
Meadows row	70	3	6-8	30-70% 1RM
Lateral raise	77	3	8-12/side	70-80% 1RM
Rainbows	188	3	10 each way	75% 1RM

Table 12.2   Full Body Power Workout 2

Exercise	Page	Sets	Reps	Load
Landmine goblet squat	82	3-5	3-5	85-90% 1RM
Landmine thruster	144	3-5	3-5	30-70% 1RM
Lateral lunge	100	3	8-12/side	70-80% 1RM
Single-arm floor press	60	3	8-12/side	70-80% 1RM
Windmills	198	3	10	75% 1RM
Landmine rollout	192	3	10	75% 1RM

Table 12.3   Cluster Set Workout

Exercise	Page	Sets	Reps	Load
Split jerk	168	3-5	2, 2, 1	85-95% 1RM
Standing two-arm landmine press	38	3-5	8-12	70-80% 1RM
Squat with sidestep	96	3	8-12/side	70-80% 1RM
Staggered single-arm row	68	3	8-12/side	70-80% 1RM
Single-arm Z press	58	3	10/side	75% 1RM
Upright row	75	3	10/side	75% 1RM

Table 12.4   Lower Body Power Workout

Exercise	Page	Sets	Reps	Load
Plyo lunge	N/A	3-5	3-5/side	30-70% 1RM
Hack squat	88	3	8-12	70-80% 1RM
Angled landmine reverse lunge	112	3	10/side	75% 1RM
Staggered RDL	128	3	8-12/side	70-80% 1RM
Lateral raise	77	3	10/side	75% 1RM
Landmine straight-leg sit-up	182	3	10	75% 1RM

ROTATIONAL POWER TRAINING

Rotational power is the generation of force around a singular axis through the integration of muscular and joint systems. Although power generation from a rotational perspective is usually more directed toward athletic performance, it can also be a challenging and engaging way to integrate power training. With regard to rotational training, it's important to have a prerequisite baseline of rotational capacity before moving into more ballistic movements. To best explain this, rotational patterns can be broken down into two main categories:

1. *Local rotational patterns*: Rotational patterns at a singular joint (i.e., external rotation of the shoulder joint)

2. *Global rotational patterns*: Rotational patterns that integrate multiple joint systems. (i.e., landmine rotational press)

Implementation of both local and global patterns is recommended. With regard to power training, global movements are generally most accepted and remain most transferable to athletic activities. See table 12.5 for a sample rotational power training workout.

Table 12.5 Rotational Power Training Workout

Exercise	Page	Sets	Reps	Load
Rotational single-arm press	46	3-5	3-5	30-70% 1RM
Landmine goblet squat	82	3-5	8-12	70-80% 1RM
Rotational squat-to-press	160	3	6-10	65-75% 1RM
Single-leg RDL	132	3	8-12	70-80% 1RM
Staggered calf raise	140	3	12/side	67-70% 1RM
Landmine march	174	3	10/side	75% 1RM

Programming for power holds many of the same principles as traditional strength training. The primary difference between strength training and power training is accomplishing the movement of weight in the shortest amount of time. Building out a program to develop more power begins with assessing the individual and keeping the program in line with their goals. Whether you are rotating, moving weight, or moving yourself, these can all be powerful movements and should be programmed specific to the intended goal. Addressing the strength, instabilities, and patterns needed can provide you with the direction needed for efficient and effective programming to become more powerful.

References

CHAPTER 1

Gottschall, J.S., J. Mills, and B. Hastings. 2013. "Integration Core Exercises Elicit Greater Muscle Activation Than Isolation Exercises." *Journal of Strength and Conditioning Research* 27 (3): 590-96. https://doi.org/10.1519/JSC.0b013e31825c2cc7.

Santana, J.C., S.M. McGill, and L.E. Brown. 2015. "Anterior and Posterior Serape." *Strength and Conditioning Journal* 37 (5): 8-13. https://doi.org/10.1519/SSC.0000000000000162.

Siff, M.C. 2002. "Functional Training Revisited." *Strength and Conditioning Journal.* 24 (5): 42-46. https://doi.org/10.1519/00126548-200210000-00011.

Tumminello, N. 2019. "The 8 Main Functional Movements." Facebook, September 28. www.facebook.com/permalink.php?/story_fbid=3076668119073674&id=176647625742419.

CHAPTER 2

Arokiasamy, P., Y. Selvamani, A.T. Jotheeswaran, and R. Sadana. 2021. "Socioeconomic Differences in Handgrip Strength and Its Association with Measures of Intrinsic Capacity Among Older Adults in Six Middle-Income Countries." *Scientific Reports* 11 (1): 19494. https://doi.org/10.1038/s41598-021-99047-9.

Bohannon, R.W. 2019. "Grip Strength: An Indispensable Biomarker for Older Adults." *Clinical Interventions in Aging.* 14: 1681-91. https://doi.org/10.2147/CIA.S194543.

CHAPTER 7

Hatfield, D.L., W.J. Kraemer, B.A. Spiering, et al. 2006. "The Impact of Velocity of Movement on Performance Factors in Resistance Exercise." *Journal of Strength and Conditioning Research* 20 (4): 760-66. https://doi.org/10.1519/R-17375.1.

Schoenfeld, B.J., J. Grgic, D. Ogborn, and J.W. Krieger. 2017. "Strength and Hypertrophy Adaptations Between Low- vs. High-Load Resistance Training: A Systematic Review and Meta-analysis." *Journal of Strength and Conditioning Research* 31 (12): 3508-23. https://doi.org/10.1519/JSC.0000000000002200.

Schoenfeld, B.J., D. Ogborn, and J.W. Krieger. 2015. "Effects of Resistance Training Frequency on Measures of Muscle Hypertrophy: A Systematic Review and Meta-analysis." *Sports Medicine* 46 (11): 1689-97. https://doi.org/10.1007/s40279-016-0543-8.

Wathen, D., T.R. Baechle, and R.W. Earle. 2008. "Periodization." In *Essentials of Strength Training and Conditioning*, 3rd ed., edited by T.R. Baechle and R.W. Earle. Human Kinetics, 511

CHAPTER 10

Pereira, P.E., Y. Motoyama, G. Esteves, et al. 2016. "Resistance Training With Slow Speed of Movement Is Better for Hypertrophy and Muscle Strength Gains Than Fast Speed of Movement." *International Journal of Applied Exercise Physiology* 5 (2): 37-43. https://doi.org/10.30472/IJAEP.V5I2.51.

Schoenfeld, B.J., J. Grgic, D. Ogborn, and J.W. Krieger. 2017. "Strength and Hypertrophy Adaptations Between Low- vs. High-Load Resistance Training: A Systematic Review and Meta-analysis." *Journal of Strength and Conditioning Research* 31 (12): 3508-23. https://doi.org/10.1519/JSC.0000000000002200.

CHAPTER 12

Filho, M.M., G.R. Venturini, O. Moreira, et al. 2022. "Effects of Different Types of Resistance Training and Detraining on Functional Capacity, Muscle Strength, and Power in Older Women: A Randomized Controlled Study." *Journal of Strength and Conditioning Research* 36 (4): 984-90. https://doi.org/10.1519/JSC.0000000000004195.

Hong, A.R., and S.W. Kim. 2018. "Effects of Resistance Exercise on Bone Health." *Endocrinology and Metabolism* (Seoul) 33 (4): 435-44. https://doi.org/10.3803/EnM.2018.33.4.435.

Stone, M.H. 1988. "Implications for Connective Tissue and Bone Alterations Resulting From Resistance Exercise Training." *Medicine and Science in Sports and Exercise* 20 (5 Suppl): S162-68. https://doi.org/10.1249/00005768-198810001-00013.

Torre, M.M., and J.-J. Temprado. 2022. "A Review of Combined Training Studies in Older Adults According to a New Categorization of Conventional Interventions." *Frontiers in Aging Neuroscience* 13: 808539. https://doi.org/10.3389/fnagi.2021.808539.

Yingling, V.R., S.L. Webb, C. Inouye, J. O, and J.J. Sherwood. 2020. "Muscle Power Predicts Bone Strength in Division II Athletes." *Journal of Strength and Conditioning Research* 34 (6): 1657-65. https://doi.org/10.1519/JSC.0000000000002222.

About the Authors

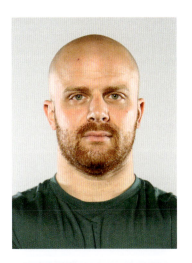

David Otey, CSCS, is an internationally recognized educator, author, and 15+ year personal trainer. Otey specializes in landmine training, unconventional training, and rotational power. He has been featured in *Men's Health*, *Muscle & Fitness*, Onnit Fitness & Nutrition, Weight Watchers, NSCA, and more. David is a graduate from Rutgers University in Exercise Physiology and was Equinox's Fitness Manager of the Year for 2015.

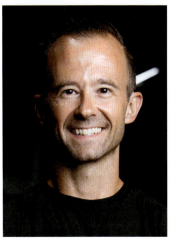

Joe Drake, ACSM-CEP, NASM-CES, CSCS, NSCA-CPT,*D, is an experienced international educator and coach with more than 15 years of experience in the fitness industry. He is the cofounder and CEO of Axiom Fitness Academy, a hands-on fitness education company offering certification courses, continuing education, and mentorship for aspiring fitness professionals. Drake has worked in nearly every aspect of the fitness industry and has served as a consultant for major industry brands such as Technogym in bringing new products to market.

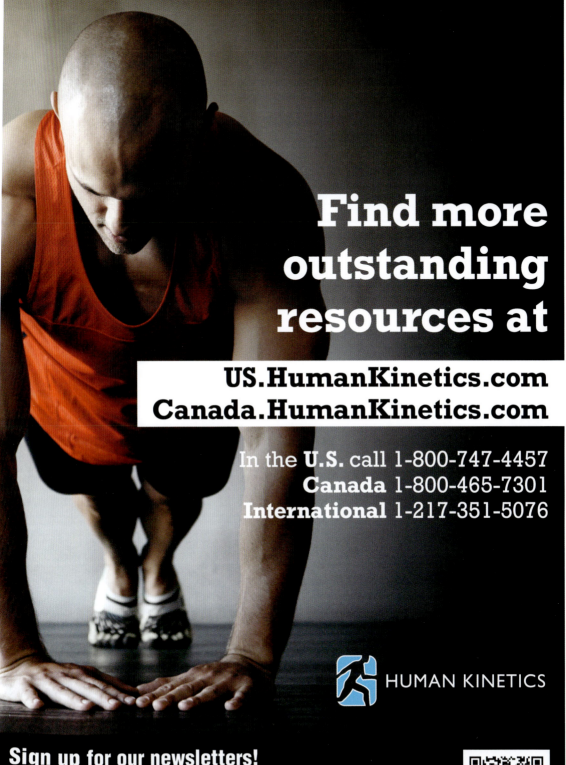

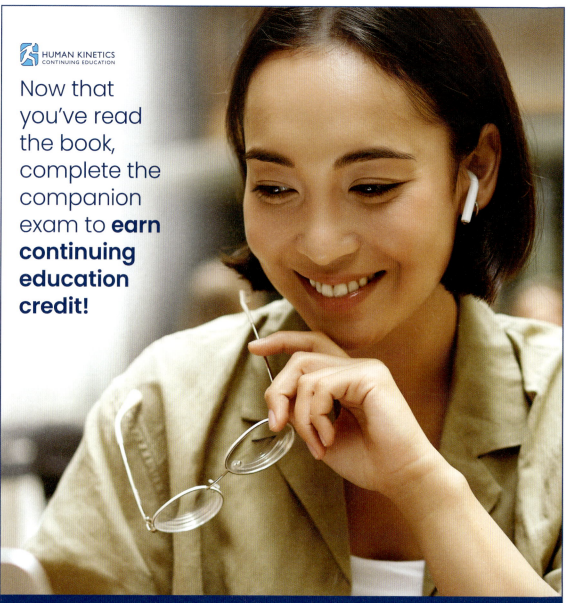
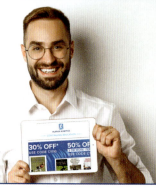